Purple Hands

A Kiwi Nurse-Midwife's Response in Times of Crisis

Barbara Walker QSO

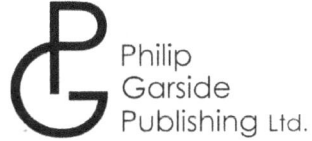

Copyright © 2020 & 2021 Barbara Walker

All rights reserved.

This book or any portion thereof may not be reproduced or used in any manner whatsoever without the express written permission of the publisher except for the use of brief quotations in a book review.

Dedicated to:
Frank and Marie Walker

Email Barbara at:
revbjwalker@xtra.co.nz

Special thanks to Wayne Blair for the author photograph and his assistance with other photographs.

Notes to readers:

To preserve their privacy, the names and identifying details of some people appearing in this book have been changed.

The views and opinions expressed in this book are the author's own and do not necessarily represent those of the people, institutions and organisations mentioned in this book.

International Print edition
Reprinted 2021
ISBN 978-1-98-857246-8

Philip Garside Publishing Ltd
PO Box 17160
Wellington 6147
New Zealand
books@pgpl.co.nz — www.pgpl.co.nz

Kindle, ePub, PDF and Audiobook editions also available

Front cover photograph:
Barbara Walker with the first baby she delivered at Las Dhure Camp, Somalia, 1980.

Contents

Foreword 7

1. First the End…Then the Beginning 9
   And then one day, everything changed 10
   An update from the police 14
2. Roots 18
   Starting out 18
   Heading north 20
   The family is complete 21
3. A Seed is Planted 21
   Challenges 22
4. Earning my Stripes 24
   I made it! 27
5. A Rocky Start 28
6. The Diameters of the Pelvis 30
7. Friendships 31
8. 'I Get My Directions from God,
   not Man…' 32
9. Mission, Marriage and Me:
   A Time to Reflect 34
10. 'You Won't Ever Make it!' 37
11. One Door Closes,
    and Another Opens Wide 38
12. Sakeo One Refugee Camp, Thailand, 1979: Baptism of Fire 39
13. Bamboo Hospitals in a Bamboo City 42
14. Another Happy Coincidence 47
15. Back to the Largest Bamboo City in the World 48
16. The Boat People: Desperation, Danger and Hope 49
17. Night Sisters, Rules, and Restrictions 53
18. Heat, Dust, Little Water, and Purple Hands 55
    An unfortunate start 55

19. Midwifery in Somalia:
    What Challenge Can Teach Us... 62
20. Wind, Rain, and Other Acts of Nature.. 65
21. Christmas in a Refugee Camp... 66
    Teach a Man to Fish….. 67
22. New Year's Eve in Nairobi, 1980... 69
23. More Adventures Await... 72
24. At the Mercy of the Banks of Africa 74
25. Up in the Air, and in God's Hands... 76
26. Farewell Somalia, Hello Calcutta 80
    Sisters of Mercy.. 81
27. Nepal... 83
28. New Directions: The World Vision Disaster Response Team 85
    Liverpool.. 86
    Going to church can be dangerous... 87
29. New Culture, New Location, New Challenges 90
    Pennell Memorial Hospital,
      North-West Frontier Province, Pakistan 90
    Bannu Beginnings 92
    If you don't ask, you won't get!... 95
30. Midwifery on the Front Line: Extraordinary Circumstances and
    Extraordinary Measures.. 96
    Questionable practice.. 96
    Neonatal Tetanus 97
    Prolapsed cords... 97
    Blood transfusions... 98
    Internal version breech extractions.. 98
    Exchange transfusions on new-born babies....................................... 99
    'Call the flying squad!' 'I AM the flying squad!' 100
    The building of a new midwifery unit 113
31. Life in Bannu... 114
32. Interlude: from Bannu to Ethiopia.. 116
    Ethiopia: First impressions.. 116
    Everyday life in the camp 119

Politics in the field 122
　　　Some time away 125
　　　An unexpected proposal..125

33. As Kiwi as… 126
　　　On the receiving end of care … 127
　　　You can take the Kiwi farm girl out of New Zealand… 130
　　　Time for self-care..132
　　　A death in the family..135
　　　Goodbye, Bannu!..136

34. Back Under African Skies: Kenya, 1988.......................... 137
　　　Kapedo Mission Hospital 140
　　　The Kenyan Nursing Council and me..................................143
　　　On the Sudanese border 149
　　　Left to die: A cultural dilemma..151

35. Zambia, via Sweden and England 152
　　　A tough decision to be made 152

36. A Fresh Beginning.. 154
　　　Zambian Nurses' Council...155
　　　The HIV and AIDS epidemic..156
　　　'A new red dress and new shoes; ready to dance for Jesus.' 157
　　　My interpreter 158
　　　A new addition to the hospital...159
　　　Stepping up to every challenge 160
　　　Resuscitating our smallest patients 161
　　　Premature babies and Kiwi ingenuity...................................161
　　　Free time in Mpongwe 162
　　　Family, friends and God 163
　　　Back to the classroom 163
　　　Moving on...164

37. Tanzania... 165
　　　Our work...166
　　　Graduation of our trained HIV/AIDS educators and counsellors...169
　　　The robbery 169
　　　University, here I come! 170
　　　Rwanda..175

    Why God, why?...175
    Traditional healers...177
    'Barbara, they want to circumcise you.'..178

38. More Challenges to Come... 179
    Return to Tanzania – HIV/AIDS Consultant for World Vision........ 180
    Family visit 180
    The truck drivers and the prostitutes 181
    Expelled from Tanzania 182
    The day a letter arrived 183
    Somalia, here I come again..183
    The day I just wanted to die..184
    The closing of one door, the opening of another..........................186
    Brunel University graduation day 186

39. Three Weeks to Learn Portuguese:
    Yeah, Right!.. 187

40. Coming Home 189
    I am safe..189
    A time of reflection..190
    Reacquaintances 190
    Re-entry 191
    Reflections 191

41. A Time for Recognition.. 195
    Fellow of the College of Nurses of Aotearoa New Zealand............... 195
    New Zealand Queen's Birthday Honours, 2000..............................196
    The Margarette Golding Award 197
    Back to my roots 197
    Rebirth of the call to ordination 198

42. 'Sister Barbara, You Still Haven't Learnt Urdu!' 200

43. A New Direction 202

Index 203

Foreword

God was with me in the vast refugee camps of Somalia and Ethiopia, on the South China Sea, in refugee camps in Thailand, in hospitals in the Afghan-Pakistan border in Kenya and Zambia, on HIV/AIDS programs in Tanzania, and in Mozambique, a land littered with landmines. Today, He continues to be with me in my work as a hospital chaplain in the Hawke's Bay Regional Hospital in New Zealand. I believe He has called me to this place for this time.

For many years, people have been asking me when I was going to write a book about my life and experiences as an international nurse-midwife aid worker. So, I have finally decided to put pen to paper and share my story with others.

I dedicate this book to the following people: Firstly, my parents, the late Frank and Marie Walker, who instilled in me the belief that we need to do our best in everything and make a difference in the lives of people we come across.

I also acknowledge the love and support of my brother and four sisters, and the many friends who have supported me along my life's journey.

Secondly, I would like to dedicate this book to the hundreds of national health workers, mainly women, and especially the traditional birth attendants, who taught me so much about midwifery in their countries, who challenged my western midwifery skills, and who gave me the title of my book; Purple Hands. I've been privileged to work with them and other national and expatriate staff in some of the world's most challenging places, learning from each other, sharing the good times, and supporting each other through the very tough and challenging times.

Over many years, I have seen the best and the worst of human beings, and I acknowledge all people, wherever they live, who are seeking to make a difference in the lives of the people they meet daily. I hope that my story will challenge other Kiwis, both young and old, to follow their call, their dreams, their passions and step out into our very needy world, taking with them their resilience, adaptability, determination, and that Kiwi number eight wire mentality. We all can make a difference in the lives of those around us, and in those in other countries, by listening, learning and sharing; but first we need to take that first step. As we come to the end of our lives, may we all be able to say, 'I sought to make a difference, and I did.'

Thirdly, I dedicate this book to my special friends the late Dr John Kerr, and his wife Dr Alison Kerr, whose support and encouragement helped make the writing of this memoir possible.

A big thank you to Dr Alison Kerr, Gail Spence, Christine Best Walker and Marie Anticich, who worked with me on this manuscript.

Finally, but most importantly, I would like to acknowledge God, my Heavenly Father, who has called me, cared for me, and journeyed with me to some of the most far-flung places in our world.

Barbara Walker

1. First the End...Then the Beginning

I left New Zealand in 1975 and didn't return to live here until 1996. I spent 20 years working overseas as a Christian aid worker, using my nursing and midwifery skills, in Australia, Vanuatu, Thailand, Somalia, Pakistan, Ethiopia, Kenya, India, Zambia, Tanzania and Mozambique. During those years, I also spent time in England, completing a variety of courses, including Tropical Medicine, Planning for Disaster, Refugee Health, and finally a master's degree in Medical Anthropology.

I returned home in 1996 because I received a death threat while in Mozambique as part of a World Vision development team. My role was to oversee the World Vision medical contribution to this programme, which was operating in the Tete region of Mozambique, in partnership with the Mozambican Ministry of Health.

I remember arriving in Mozambique in January 1996 and driving through the city of Tete and seeing a surprising number of people with only one leg or no legs, using crutches. I asked Rashid, the World Vision team leader who had collected me from the airport, what had happened. He explained this was because thousands of Mozambican citizens had been severely injured by accidentally stepping on the thousands of landmines laid throughout Mozambique during the civil war. Hundreds more had been killed by landmines. Specialised demining teams were working in Mozambique, trying to locate the land mines and defuse them. In 2015, Mozambique was declared free of land mines with over 171,100 land mines having been removed.

Let me share some background on Mozambique: The Portuguese sailor Vasco de Gama arrived in Mozambique in 1498 and a gradual process of colonisation took place over the next 500 or so years. In 1962, exiled activists met in Tanzania to form the Mozambique Liberation Front, Frelimo, headed by Eduardo Mondlane. In 1964, Frelimo forces started a war of independence and in 1975 Mozambique finally gained its independence. The Frelimo party ruled under a single party system when Samora Machel, the leader of the Frelimo party became president. In 1976, Renamo, an anti-Frelimo resistance group, was set up by Rhodesian officers, and clashes began to occur with the Frelimo in Mozambique. From 1977 to 1992 there was ongoing civil war between Frelimo and

Renamo. In 1986, the Mozambican President Samora Machel was killed in an unexplained plane crash in South Africa. Fighting ended in 1992 and the country's first multi-party elections were held in 1994. In 1995 Mozambique joined the British Commonwealth. An estimated one million Mozambicans died in the fighting or from starvation during the civil war.

My home for the next two years was to be Tete, a city of over 1 million people, on the Zambezi river in the Tete province of Mozambique. Tete was over 1,000 kilometres from Maputo, the capital city of Mozambique, where the World Vision National office was located. Harare, the capital of Zimbabwe was only 338 kilometres away, so it was easier to go and buy supplies there rather than driving for days to Maputo.

I was working with a seven-member team of expat, experienced aid workers and a team of Mozambican nationals, including medical staff, logistics staff, agricultural staff, drivers and guards. Given my inability to learn foreign languages (despite a three-week course in Portuguese), I was thrilled to find that John, administrator of the World Vision Mozambique medical program, was fluent in English. He also had a wealth of knowledge and was very willing to guide me in all aspects of the culture, language and history of Mozambique, as well as giving me the background of the World Vision medical programme which we would be working together on.

I lived in a small, two-bedroom house on a World Vision compound in Tete, along with five other WV workers who lived in other houses on the compound. The compound had a high fence around it, with armed guards. Our team leader Rashid and his wife, both from India, lived nearby in another small compound.

And then one day, everything changed

My world turned upside down one Saturday morning in June 1996. I was sitting at my dining-table, drinking a leisurely cup of coffee and planning activities for the coming weeks. I had been in the country six months and was enjoying working with the World Vision Mozambique medical team, as together we were planning to address some of the major health concerns facing the Tete regions: ongoing and increasing malnutrition, the need to re-establish vaccination programs after 17 years of civil war, and the need to upskill local staff, who had gone through many years of a brutal civil war. There was also a huge need to teach mothers how to read and write, which was the focus of one of the programs that I was involved in.

My Saturday morning, usually a time for rest and relaxation after a busy week, was interrupted by a loud knock at the door. I found the armed guard who protected our compound standing there. 'Bom dia,' (Good morning in Portuguese) he said, to which I replied, 'Bom dia,' as he handed me a white envelope.

'Obrigado,' (thank you), I said, shutting the door. I sat down to open the letter; handwritten on a single sheet of white paper were the following words:

> 'Unless you and your senior Mozambican staff raise the salaries of the Mozambique health staff, you and your senior Mozambican staff will be killed at the end of the year.'

'Surely this is a joke!' I thought. Stunned, I read and re-read the letter. Why would someone send me a death threat? I had felt truly called by God to work alongside Mozambican people and help rebuild their medical programmes after years of civil war. I was also aware that many Mozambicans held the perception that all expatriates had money. World Vision, along with several international aid agencies, meet regularly to discuss wages for local staff to ensure that what they were being paid was fair, depending on the different work they were involved in.

So, why was I being targeted when I wasn't the one who set the salaries of staff? Suddenly, I felt very alone in this war-ravaged country. Thoughts were racing through my mind. My emotions ran high. I felt angry, fearful, anxious, and worried, all at the same time. Had I offended someone? A thousand and one thoughts began swirling around in my mind. I needed to talk to someone; I decided to show the letter to my expatriate colleague Anne, who lived next door. I knocked on her door and she welcomed me in. 'Read this,' I said, shoving the letter at her. She looked at me, realizing that this was serious. Anne's mouth fell open as she read the message. 'Oh, Barbara,' she said, 'This is awful!' giving me a reassuring hug. We sat in silence, trying to decide what to do. 'Let's drive over to Rashid's place and show him the letter,' Anne suggested. (Rashid and his wife lived nearby on another small World Vision compound.)

Our land cruiser was parked on our compound, and we asked the driver to take us to Rashid's house. A few minutes later, we arrived at their house and were duly invited in. Rashid and Anika sat us down and offered us a cold drink, before asking, 'What can we do for you?' Wordlessly, I passed the letter to Rashid. Glancing at me questioningly, he took the note. A look of shock crossed his face and he came over and hugged me. 'I am sorry, Barbara, that you have received this. We will support you through this, I promise.' I knew he would, but suddenly I felt panicky and tearful. The threat was beginning to feel very real. 'I'll increase security on the compound and inform the World Vision National director in Maputo,' Rashid assured me. 'And I'll contact the local police.' After a time of prayer, the driver took Anne and me back to the compound.

The following night, at our weekly expat staff meeting, Rashid informed our seven-member team of the death threat. As a senior member of the World Vision team, John was also invited to come that night. We decided that this situation would remain within the four walls of the house and wouldn't be discussed amongst the local staff. Rashid urged us to be vigilant and to report any concerns to him without delay. My colleagues rallied around me, offering their support and the evening ended with prayer. I struggled to sleep that night and for many months to come. The smallest noise unnerved me, and I never felt safe.

Questions tormented me: Did one of the medical team write the letter? Or was it someone who had a grudge against World Vision? It wasn't only directed at me but also at our senior Mozambican staff – why? Would they really carry out the threat? And if so, how? Waves of fear washed over me. I became suspicious of everyone and my nerves were frayed. It was also very hard for John, as he was the most senior Mozambican staff member on our team. The death threat included him as well.

On the Monday following that eventful Saturday morning, Rashid and John went to see the Tete chief of police and informed him of the note. A few days later, he came to see me and asked for names of possible suspects. John was present at the meeting. I thought about it, felt that a reply could place me in even more danger, and refused to supply a list of names. After some discussion, it was decided that the police would interview all World Vision Mozambican medical staff over the coming days. The police chief who had come to see me asked us to provide writing pads, pens and a light bulb before the interviews could start. He explained that such supplies were needed to conduct the interviews. I could understand the pads and pens, but the light bulb? He explained that the light bulb in room that they would be using for the interviews had broken and they didn't have the money to buy a replacement. This didn't exactly fill me with confidence.

Despite all of this, both John and I continued to lead the medical team. I found the weekly team meetings very hard as we discussed the upcoming work plans; still the question haunted me: 'Which one of you wrote the death threat?' Weeks ticked by, and the police seemed to have lost interest in my case. When Rashid asked the police for an update, they told him the case was ongoing. Soon, months had ticked by.

In my many years as a humanitarian relief worker, I had never broken a contract, and I desperately wanted to continue in my role as manager of the World Vision medical programme and complete the projects in Mozambique. But with the death threat hanging over me, I felt uncertain. As the months passed and I became increasingly conscious that the end of the year was looming, tension mounted, accompanied by unhurried police investigations. But I forced myself to be patient and work with the police, as I was a guest in their country, after all. I didn't write home to my parents about this situation as I didn't want to worry them.

John and I continued to work with the team, and I spent time travelling with the Mozambique staff, visiting the various World Vision feeding centres which had been set up in some of the poorer areas of Tete province. Because these feeding centres were in very remote areas, access to them was limited due to roads near the feeding centres not yet having been cleared of land mines. To visit one such feeding centre, we had to cross over the border into Malawi then drive the length of Malawi, and cross back into Tete province to access a major mine-free road to the feeding centre. If we were late in reaching the border crossing, we had to sleep at the border in our land cruisers. This happened on more than one occasion. Many of the clinics I oversaw were on the more minor roads, which may or may not have been checked yet by the demining teams. As these teams cleared each road, signs would be erected on the side of the road informing everyone that the road was safe. So, we relied on the driver to ensure that these roads had been demined. A lot of the travel that I did was in very remote areas and if we had a toilet stop, we didn't wander off into the bushes on the side of the road as we couldn't be sure if that area had been checked for landmines! This added to the excitement of the work, to say the least.

An update from the police

After several months, the local police finally got back to Rashid and me, informing us they had interviewed all the staff members and hadn't found the letter writer. They said the only way to find out was to arrest them all and beat a confession out of them. This seemed barbaric to me; perhaps this was something that happened in this part of the world, but I chose to say no. The next comment from the Police chief absolutely astounded me, 'You're the only person we haven't interviewed,' he declared, and ordered me to come to the station the following morning for an interview. 'You must be joking,' I thought. I complied, insisting that John needed to be with me for any interview, as I didn't have enough Portuguese.

The Police chief met us at the station the next morning. 'I want to interview you alone,' he informed me. 'Come with me to the interview room.' 'I need my colleague John to come with me and translate,' I insisted. 'I have very little Portuguese and I need John.' The Police chief refused point blank. 'You must come with me alone,' he stated slightly raising his voice. We had reached a stalemate. Again, I told him I wouldn't be interviewed without John. The Police chief and John started a dialogue in Portuguese. I couldn't understand a word they said but it was obvious that neither of them was prepared to back down. The Police chief was furious and again ordered me to come with him. I looked at my colleague with tear-filled eyes and refused to move. The Police chief stormed off, uttering a few angry words. John and I were driven back to the World Vision office which was on the edge of town, and there I met with our team leader, Rashid. We discussed what do to next. We obviously weren't going to get any more help from the police.

I had conflicting emotions and felt ambivalent. When I arrived in Mozambique, I had signed a two-year contract, and here I was, wanting to walk away from the job after just six months. I also didn't want to let down the people of New Zealand, who so generously supported the work of World Vision in Mozambique by donating money and supporting events like the annual 40 Hour Famine. I had spoken to the New Zealand High Commissioner who was based in Harare, Zimbabwe, about a project which I was hoping to start in a very poor part of Tete Province.

We wanted to set up a project that involved gathering women and their young toddlers together, feeding the children with high energy porridge, and running literacy classes for the women, which would include reading and writing. He was very supportive of this project and helped fund it. I hated the thought of abandoning this and other projects I'd initiated.

Another project which I was involved in, involved investing in the Mozambican World Vision staff. Mozambique had joined the British Commonwealth in 1995, and there was a huge interest in learning English. Our staff were very keen to learn, and I had arranged for Nick and Lucy (the grown children of Sheila and Roger, friends from Liverpool) to come and teach.

Despite my worry over the project's future, having Nick and Lucy staying with me helped to take my mind off the death threat hanging over me. As time passed, the end of the year was coming closer and the storm clouds seemed to grow larger and blacker. I wasn't coping well, and I knew something had to change. I had to wonder whether, if I left, the projects I had set up would continue, or if all my efforts would be wasted. I forced myself to go to work each day, commit to these projects, and patiently wait for the police to come up with something.

By early November, the situation was becoming untenable. I was losing sleep at night and felt it couldn't trust anyone. The letter had said I would be killed by the end of the year unless senior staff received a pay increase; the end of the year was only one month away.

Things turned around after I phoned World Vision New Zealand director, Colin Prentice. He rang Bruce McConchie, a fellow New Zealander who was then the Director of World Vision Southern Africa. I felt somewhat relieved when Colin suggested that I give Bruce a ring. Bruce and I had worked together in Tanzania; he knew me well, and he knew that I was someone who was normally very strong, having gone through some tough times during my aid worker journey. Later that day I phoned and shared with him what had happened. Bruce voiced his concerns about the death threat that I had received and on-going stress it was causing me and asked me to come to South Africa to meet with him. He made arrangements for this to happen, and the next day, a Friday, I was driven to Harare and flown to South Africa. Bruce met me at Johannesburg, and we went to the World Vision office. He listened quietly as I explained the situation and finally said, 'Barbara, we need to get you out of Mozambique as quickly as possible.'

We developed a plan. I was to fly back to Harare on Saturday; the World Vision driver would collect me and drive me back to Tete and I would go to work on Monday morning as if nothing had happened. The expats on the team would be informed, but not the Mozambican staff, which included John. I really struggled with this decision as we had worked so closely together but I felt I needed to abide by what Bruce had arranged. On Monday morning, I went to the office and continued with my work, hoping no-one would notice my inner turmoil. I knew I had to leave Mozambique for my own safety and sanity, but it was an incredibly hard thing to do. Working in African countries, I'd learnt that farewells were extremely important as they gave the person leaving a chance to say good-bye and to ask forgiveness for any wrongs they had done, and vice versa. Now I was leaving without saying goodbye. Walking out on John and the team felt like a betrayal; I knew he would be hurt, as I would be if the situation was reversed.

I left the office late afternoon and climbed into the waiting land cruiser. My heart ached as we entered the compound gate for the very last time. I walked into my house and found that Mary, my house girl, had just finished preparing my dinner. I thanked her and signalled I didn't require dinner tomorrow night as I was going out. She probably thought I was going out to one of my colleague's home for dinner, but I knew I was going out, and leaving Mozambique, never to return. Mary said goodbye and left the house. I never saw Mary again. I ate the dinner she'd prepared and started to pack my one suitcase. I fought back the tears, as I was sad to be leaving, but also relieved, knowing, as I did every moment of every day, that the end of the year was fast approaching. Later that evening, my expatriate colleagues came to say goodbye, and they kindly sent my belongings back to New Zealand some months later.

I spent a restless night trying to process the events of the last few months. When I'd arrived in Mozambique, I'd decided this would possibly be my last overseas assignment. After nearly 20 years of relief and development work overseas, frequently in desperate conditions and coping daily with suffering and despair, I'd begun to think seriously about heading back to New Zealand. Working in such tough conditions over so many years had taken its toll on me physically, emotionally, mentally and spiritually. But I had no idea what I would do or how would I adjust to life back in New Zealand. So many questions. My faith in God was a bit shaky just then. Walking away without completing my contract was gut-wrenching. I'd never broken a contract before and felt I'd somehow failed. Not being able to say goodbye and thank people was even tougher. Many times, I asked God, 'Why?' I was deeply distressed that God's early call for me to be a nurse-midwife aid worker was ending this way.

At 6.00 the following morning, my driver arrived as planned. I loaded my one suitcase in the vehicle and was driven to Harare. From there I flew to London to stay with friends, Pat and Jean. Pat had spent several years working in Afghanistan as a nurse-midwife but was now a mission director living in England. We had first met in Bannu, Pakistan many years earlier, and she had extensive experience in providing support to people who had had similar experiences to mine; I trusted her and respected her wisdom and guidance. I also really appreciated the pastoral and spiritual support she gave me then before I began my journey home. Because I was employed by World Vision International at this time, I was asked to fly home via the World Vision International Head Office in California, where I met with World Vision staff experienced in counselling and support. I also spent time with the World Vision Security Team, who reviewed what had happened, and looked at what could have been done differently. I was advised not to return to Mozambique.

Some weeks later, I returned to New Zealand, still traumatised by these events. My return signalled the end of my career as nurse-midwife aid worker. Just as I arrived back in New Zealand, Sheryl Thayer, a Red Cross nurse from Southland, was killed in Chechnya just shy of her 40th birthday. 'There but for the grace of God go I,' I thought. Since I left Mozambique in 1996, six expats have been killed there. Some were workers, some were visitors. Until the 1990s, aid workers were rarely killed, but today this is becoming increasingly common as mercenaries, insurgents and political activists realise they can use aid workers to put pressure on governments and gain publicity for their cause. Previously, aid workers had a kind of diplomatic immunity because they were going into desperate situations and laying down their lives for people in need. Whenever I hear of another aid worker being killed, I shudder and think, 'Why wasn't it me?' and I quietly thank God it wasn't.

When I came home, I wondered, if I could have done something differently and what would have happened if I'd stayed. Did I overreact to the death threat? Hindsight is very useful, and I can look back now and know deep down that leaving Mozambique at that time was the right decision for me. As I jumped into the land cruiser that day in November 1996, I left that country knowing that by working in partnership with the Mozambican Ministry of Health, with the wonderful support from my colleague John, we did make a difference in the lives of some people.

I returned to New Zealand exhausted. Nearly 21 years of working in what was often very challenging and heart-breaking situations had taken its toll. I needed time just to be, time to spend time with my family, especially getting to know new members of my family who had arrived while I was away, time with my friends who had supported me over those years, but most importantly, time just to be still and acknowledge and give thanks to God. He had been with me throughout my journey, from when I was a 13-year-old country girl, and as a new journey began to unfold for me in New Zealand, I trusted Him to guide me into this next stage of my life.

So how did this New Zealand girl, born in a small town in 1951, end up getting a death threat and being evacuated out of Mozambique in 1996? To find out, I invite you to travel with me on my journey as the story unfolds.

2. Roots

Starting out

My life began in Riverton, a small fishing village at the bottom of New Zealand's South Island. I am told my birth was induced because Mum's doctor wanted to ensure I was safely delivered before he went on holiday. I can understand this. But years later, working as a midwife in remote places all around the world, I learnt very quickly that babies arrive when they are ready, despite any inconvenience it might cause.

I was born on the 9th of August 1951, my paternal grandfather Vaughan Walker's birthday, and was christened in the beautiful historic Anglican church there. Desperately wanting a son, my father had chosen the name Richard Llewelyn, but when I arrived, the name was quickly changed to Barbara Judith.

My parents were Frank, a teacher at Riverton Primary School, and Marie Walker, a home science teacher. As our family grew, mum became a fulltime mother, her teaching career put on hold. My sister Wendy was two then, and our maternal grandparents, Mabel and Frank de la Perrelle

(Gaga), also lived in Riverton, where Gaga was manager of the Bank of New Zealand.

We left Riverton when I was four years old, and by then Wendy and I had a younger sister named Susan. We headed north in my parents' car to the small coal-mining town of Millerton on the West Coast of the South Island. My father was appointed headmaster of Millerton Primary School, and Gaga became manager of the Bank of New Zealand in Westport, the nearest shopping centre, about 60 minutes away. I started my schooling at Millerton Primary, which at the time had about 20 pupils. My father was the only teacher.

Millerton was situated high up on the hills above a small village called Granity, with a very steep, winding, gravel road the only link between the two places. It was a fascinating place to live in: Everything was centred around what was happening at the coal mine and just about everyone and everything in town was connected with it – miners and their families, the mine support staff, the few local shop keepers, and of course, the school. I remember watching miners walk up the road in the early mornings, carrying their lunch boxes and returning late afternoon, tired after a tough day's work underground, ready to have an early dinner and an early night. Although they may have had a tough day, they also looked clean, having bathed in the large bath houses which were found at the mine. Some days, a siren pierced the air, and we knew there'd been an accident in the mine. Families would immediately migrate to the mine gates and anxiously wait for news. Few Millerton people owned cars and getting transport to the main business centre of Westport was difficult. Luckily, there was a daily bus which was often full of locals, heading into Westport to carry out their business.

Our house in Millerton was an old wooden villa with three bedrooms and several coal fires for heating. The toilet was outside at the back of the house and the small, detached building contained just a wooden bench with a hole in it, with a metal can underneath. The local 'night man' was able to access the can from the back of the wooden bench, and every couple of days he came to collect the full can and replace it with another. Our toilet had a light, along with lots of spiders, so it wasn't a place to spend a long time in. Constantly during my later relief and disaster work, I was reminded just what luxury we had in Millerton! In the field, 'toilets' ranged from DIY pit latrines, to blocked toilets, to none!

During our three years in Millerton, two more girls, Jillian and Jennifer, were born into our family.

Heading north

We left the South Island, known to the locals as 'the Mainland' of New Zealand, when I was eight years old, and headed north to the province of Taranaki on the North Island's west coast. There, Dad was appointed headmaster of a two-teacher school in the small farming community of Mokoia, a tiny township twenty minutes from the town of Hawera. Mokoia boasted three churches; Anglican, Catholic and Presbyterian, a general store, and a large dairy factory which processed milk into cheese. Mokoia Primary School was the centre of the community and the arrival of Mr and Mrs Walker and their five daughters boosted school numbers greatly. For many of my primary school years, my father was my teacher. This was tough sometimes because he was probably stricter on us to avoid showing favouritism. Also, we were encouraged to be models of good behaviour to the other children, which was a lot to expect of five active young girls!

I needed friendships away from my sisters at times, and a girl called Anne became my close friend in Mokoia. I spent many happy times playing with her and helping her father Clarrie on their large sheep farm. Clarrie and I would spend hours walking in rain, hail, or shine to check on the sheep, especially at lambing time, and I loved the freedom I found on the farm. He taught me much about sheep farming and lambing and allowed me to deliver complicated cases. I was very keen to learn everything he could teach me, and I became quite skilled.

Occasionally, we came across a birthing ewe with a lamb's back leg protruding from her rear, and Clarrie would guide me through the process of inserting my arm inside the ewe and gently locating the lamb's two front feet. By placing the front feet on either side of the lamb's head, and carefully pulling, I successfully delivered several live lambs. Little did I know that years later, I would use similar techniques in Pakistan, on women who arrived at our hospital in advanced labour with babies who had already died in utero (the option of carrying out a caesarean for a deceased baby was not an option). I loved spending time on Clarrie's family farm, dreaming about marrying a farmer, and settling down to help run a large sheep station, somewhere in New Zealand. Sadly, this hasn't happened, at least not yet!

The family is complete

In 1961, my dad became the teaching headmaster at Portland Primary School, just south of Whangarei, in Northland. It was sad to leave Mokoia, my friend Anne, and the farm, but dad loaded up our Morris Oxford car and headed north. My family was used to a life with five girls, and with the youngest now eight, we assumed our family was complete. But one day, our parents told us we were going to have another baby. My dad had always wanted a son so badly that before we girls were born, he would choose boys' names: no scans existed in those days. I often wonder if he had given up hope and chosen a girl's name this time around. When Mum went into labour, Dad dropped her at the maternity suite at Whangarei Hospital and came home. A few hours later, the phone rang, and we heard Dad talking. Suddenly, he began to cry. We were shocked – we'd never seen Dad cry. 'What's wrong?' we asked when he put down the phone.

Wiping away his tears, Dad said, 'We have a son! You girls have a baby brother.' We were so excited we got on our bikes and rode around the town yelling, 'We've got a baby brother!' News spread quickly and the whole town was thrilled for the Walkers. Dad took us to the hospital to meet our new brother, who was named Philip, after his maternal grandfather, and Vaughan after his paternal grandfather. Our family was indeed complete.

3. A Seed is Planted

Dad came from a Methodist family, but he had never been christened. Because Mum and we kids had all been christened Anglican, one day Dad decided it was time for him to take the plunge. We children knew how babies were christened; the vicar picked up the baby up and poured water over its head. How would the vicar hold Dad in his arms? Our minds boggled. When Dad's Christening Day arrived, we were most disappointed when the minister simply reached up and poured water on Dad's hair.

Attending church services was a regular part of most people's lives in those days, and as a family we attended the local Anglican Church and Sunday school in the community where we lived. During the school holidays, some of the local churches would host camps for school children. One year, I attended a Christian school holiday camp at Whangarei Heads, run by the headmaster and his wife from a nearby school.

This camp was life-changing; there I met God in a deeply personal way. One morning after the morning speaker had finished giving his message, he invited those of us who would like to dedicate their lives to following Christ to come forward for prayer. I responded and went forward to the front of the stage. As the speaker prayed for me, I felt strongly that God was calling me to become a missionary nurse, aid worker.

I remember going home, where Mum was feeding my wee brother. I shared with her that I had become a Christian and wanted to become a missionary nurse. She said, 'That's nice, dear, but you're young and have plenty of time to make up your mind.' I wasn't to be so easily put off! The call to be a missionary nurse has stayed with me all my life and I have obeyed that call. Later, when things got tough overseas and I felt incredibly lonely, and yes, in danger, I would recall that holiday camp, where God met with me and I met with Him. It's possible that God had always had this plan for me, but until then I was too young to hear Him. Many years after this, my grandmother Mabel shared a memory with me: She said that when I was just a little girl, she noticed that I would sit at attention during church services, completely focused on the minister. I wonder if I was thinking even then that I wanted to be a minister of God too, something I would indeed become, later in life.

Challenges

During my primary schooling, Dad was usually my classroom teacher as well as being the headmaster. As I've said, being the headmaster's child was tough because the expectations not only from Mum and Dad, but also from the community, were high; headmaster's kids, vicar's kids and policemen's kids were all expected to behave.

Expectations to achieve academically were high, too, especially among five capable girls, all born close together. I felt I had to run to keep up with my sisters; I always considered them to be much brighter than I was. However, I didn't speak to anyone about this. I kept to myself, and kept a stiff upper lip, as was the way, but I knew I was different. I was born into a family of readers, but I really struggled with reading and thought reading was a waste of time. At times, I thought people who read were rude! I would much rather be doing something active outside than sitting down reading a book. Even worse, although Susan my next sister was two years younger, I worried that she would catch up with me and be in the same class, or even pass me. This was a huge fear for me that I internalized and continued to say nothing about to anyone. I struggled with this throughout my schooling and it wasn't until many years later that I would be diagnosed with dyslexia.

In 1965, I left Portland Primary School and started at Whangarei Girls High School. A short time later Dad was appointed as headmaster at Ohaupo School. Ohaupo was a small farming community south of Hamilton in the middle of the North Island. I attended the nearest high school which was Melville High School.

I was sure that God had a hand in my going there; the school was led by fine Christian teachers and had a strong Christian student group. A teacher named Alison, who was also my hockey and cricket coach, led the Crusader Group, a Christian student club. Several of her friends were missionary nurses overseas and she invited them to speak to our group. I was so touched by their stories that I asked if I could sign up then and there! I was impatient that I had to keep learning and training but came to realise that training was part of God's preparation. I needed to trust in Him and accept His perfect timing.

I enjoyed my time at Melville High School, although I continued to struggle with schoolwork. I managed to pass School Certificate, knowing it was important if I wanted to become a missionary nurse. I persevered, and the following year I managed to get my University Entrance accredited, which was a huge shock to everyone, myself included. My parents didn't believe me when I told them, but of course they were pleased.

I've always wondered whether I was accredited because the staff wanted me to take on a role within the student leadership; despite my best efforts my marks during the year were far from brilliant! The staff asked my parents to allow me to come back and be Head Girl for my final year, which I did. This gave me some time to grow up and mature and think about my future. My desire to become a nurse and serve overseas continued to grow, and without telling anyone, I sent away for the application form to apply to Nursing at Greenlane Hospital in Auckland. My parents were puzzled when an envelope addressed to me came from Greenlane Hospital and I had to do some fast talking when I got home. In the end, they helped me fill in the papers. Deep down I knew that nursing was the right course for me, and I think they did, too.

4. Earning my Stripes

God's plans for my life were continuing to unfold. I was duly accepted into the nursing programme at Greenlane Hospital, which would start in January 1970. In those days it was compulsory to stay in the nurses' home by the hospital, and I began my training with a class of 30 girls. Academically, I knew nursing was going to be a challenge for me. But I also knew that God had called me, and 'When He calls, He equips.' So, I trusted Him to get me through.

I loved my nursing training. I completed my six weeks prelim nurse course and then started on the wards as a student nurse. As student nurses, we wore white paper caps and white uniforms, and the number of stripes on the shoulder area on our uniforms signified how senior we were. As a first-year nurse, I had just one stripe on each shoulder; student nurses were on the second to bottom rung of the ladder (and scrubbing bed pans was a regular part of our job). Other reminders of our position included the veil-wearing matron who looked so stern when she visited the wards; consultants in three-piece suits who arrived with an entourage of registrars, house officers and students; and the ward sisters whose eagle eyes saw everything that was going on. When the daily troop of consultants arrived each day, my colleagues and I were encouraged to look, listen and learn but not to get in the way. We accepted this as part of the process.

My inexperience was made clear on several occasions. A few weeks after my preliminary studies had been completed, I was on afternoon shift in a medical ward. An elderly man had died, and the senior nurse asked me to help her lay him out. Although I'd never seen a dead person before, I bravely agreed. Gathering a wash bowl, clean linen, aprons and gloves, we entered the room. The man was lying flat on the bed and was still warm. The nurse explained that we would wash him and place him in a shroud for the funeral directors to collect him. We started the process in silence.

'Now, we're going to roll him over,' the nurse said. I gently pushed the body towards her, and gasped when the man made a groaning noise! I completely lost my nerve and was ready to fly out of that door, and out of nursing! It took some fast talking by the nurse to keep me in the room, explaining that the noise was probably just trapped air, and a normal occurrence. I've never forgotten that incident – one of many that shocked me but put me in good stead for my nursing career to follow. Little did I know then that in years to come, I would be witness to hundreds of deaths in more than fourteen countries around the world. I saw people die in hospitals, under trees, in mud huts, in the back of trucks, floating down rivers, on operating tables and in my arms.

Death will come to us all one day, and I am still deeply moved to be with someone who is dying. The barriers of language, race and religion aren't important at that time. It's just one human supporting another. I hope and trust that when my time comes, there will be another human being there to be with me.

Another memorable encounter with death occurred later, when I was a registered nurse, working at Greenlane Hospital. At morning teatime, I sent the nursing staff off for their break, leaving a couple of hospital aides to manage the 30-bed ward with me. A very tall man who had been ill with cancer for some time had died, the paperwork had been completed, and we were to wash him before the funeral director arrived. To speed things up, I decided to wash the patient myself. I entered his room and I rolled him towards me so I could wash his back. Suddenly, I lost my balance, fell on the floor and the deceased man fell on top of me. I lay on my back, shocked and feeling stupid. I couldn't reach the bell, and I didn't want to scream for help in case a patient came in and found me. My plan had certainly backfired. Waiting for my colleagues to return from morning tea was the longest wait I've ever endured. It was a very awkward position to be in and I felt a bit of an idiot. I was helpless and just had to be patient; the staff would return, but not soon enough!

They finally returned and someone called, 'Staff Nurse Walker, where are you?' 'I'm in here,' I yelled out, 'Please open the door and come in.' But no-one heard me. Time passed. Then I heard a knock and a nurse came in. The look on her face said it all. Other nurses came in and stared in shocked horror. But they couldn't move the dead man; he was too heavy. They raced off to fetch some hospital orderlies. I continued to lie in this very awkward position. Finally, the orderlies arrived, and it took four of them to lift the deceased man off me and onto the bed. Then they pulled me to my feet with stunned looks on their faces. As they left, my nursing colleagues said, 'We'll take over. I think you deserve your coffee break.' I didn't argue. I realised that laying out someone alone was not one of my brighter ideas, and I never did it again. Although the incident was never mentioned, I'm sure I was a target for some black hospital humour.

Part of a nurse's training is to develop the skills needed to work with the public, often to protect our patients, and I took this part of my role seriously. In the 1970s, Greenlane Hospital was a major heart hospital in New Zealand, a busy place with an international reputation. Patients from all over New Zealand were flown in for heart surgery, including new-born babies. The cardiac surgeons and the cardiac nurses were an amazing group of people dedicated to improving the lives of New Zealanders through ground-breaking surgery. The chief cardiac surgeon was an impressive man. I met him one Saturday morning when I was a second-year nurse working on one of the cardiac wards. I was standing by the nurses' desk with the patients' charts beside me when this casually dressed man approached and started to look at the patients' charts. 'Excuse me,' I said. 'These charts are confidential.' He smiled and said, 'Well done nurse, for questioning me. We haven't met. I am Mr Barratt-Boyes, the head cardiac surgeon here.' (He later became Sir Brian Barratt-Boyes). I smiled back, wishing the ground would swallow me up.

My first cardiac arrest case was in a women's medical ward. Such an event is always traumatic. We had been trained in what to do but it isn't until there is an actual live situation where the team is fighting hard to save a person's life that the seriousness kicks in. This patient had had a good night's sleep and was now asking for a bed pan. She was on strict bed rest, so I pulled the curtains and helped her to get onto the pan. I passed her the bell and waited just outside. Suddenly I heard a strange noise. When I opened the curtains, I found her collapsed and looking a horrible colour. Although I was a junior nurse, I was aware of the emergency. I rang the bell three times. It was a full-on emergency.

Staff arrived and ordered me to do cardiac massage while they inserted a drip and started mouth-to-mouth on her. This woman's life literally lay in the balance as we worked to save her. It was an incredibly tense situation. Thankfully, because of the specialised treatment available at that time, she came around and was transferred to the Coronary Care Unit, and a few days later, was back on the ward. It was lovely to see her, and she was delighted to be alive. Her only complaint was that she had very sore ribs. Every nurse remembers their first death and their first cardiac arrest.

We also hang on to kind words and encouragement. I well remember the day I got my ward report after my first six weeks as a student nurse on the Ear, Nose and Throat ward. Ward Sister Anne, called me into her office and handed me my report: 'It is a good report nurse, you've done well. Keep up the good work! You have the makings of a good nurse. Don't let me down!'

Her words 'Don't let me down!' often came to mind as I continued my nursing career in places so incredibly different from my hospital training at Greenlane and helped me to carry on.

I made it!

Although my training didn't involve specialities such as orthopaedics or psychiatric nursing, by the time I came to sit my state final exams I found I had enough knowledge on which to build my nursing practice. I had found the nursing course theory difficult but enjoyed interacting with the patients and their families and the practical aspect of nursing. I loved the medical and surgical wards, finding the technical side of specialised areas like Intensive Care and Coronary Care a bit too complex for me. During my three-year course, I also completed maternity training, which provided basic knowledge for my plans to do midwifery training.

After three years of training, I was delighted to find I had passed the state finals. It was a proud night when I walked across the stage at the Auckland Town Hall to receive my New Zealand Registered Nurse's medal and certificate. My parents, grandmother, and young brother joined me for this milestone. I was one step nearer my calling to become a missionary nurse. After graduation, I completed a one-year post-graduate programme in infectious diseases and complicated wounds wards. Once again, this would provide valuable experience for the years that followed.

5. A Rocky Start

It was coming up to Easter, 1974 and I had a few weeks free between finishing my staffing year at Greenlane Hospital and starting my midwifery course. Excited to get started, my friend Mary and I contacted a missionary nurse who was the matron of a small mission hospital on Ambae Island, north of Port Vila in the New Hebrides (now known as Vanuatu) and offered our services. Mary and I flew into Port Vila, staying a few nights at the local hospital, and then caught a flight to the small island of Ambae, which was to be our home for the next six weeks. The island's community included several expatriates, a school, a large Anglican church and a well-constructed but basically equipped hospital.

Soon after our arrival, a woman came to the hospital with labour difficulties; Matron Betty decided to transfer her to the larger island of Santo, where the hospital had facilities for caesarean sections. The only way to get the labouring woman there was by fishing boat, so Mary and I accompanied the patient on the journey, along with two experienced local midwives from the hospital, and crew members who knew the way. It was late afternoon when we left. As we headed out of the bay and turned in the direction of Santo Island, the boat was ploughing along, and the woman was doing well.

After some hours, the weather changed, the wind came up and the boat was tossed about on the waves. The fishing boat had no life jackets, radio, or flares and Mary and I began to worry. Suddenly, the engine died, the boat began to rock violently, and the crew rushed around looking extremely worried. By now the woman was in strong labour with severe pain. The midwives cared for her as best they could, with limited pain relief and increasing worry.

Mary and I were distracted from our own worry when a loud scratching noise started to come from a drawer in the room where the woman lay. Huge waves crashing over the deck continued to toss the boat about as I slowly made my way to the drawer, gripping the furniture to steady myself. I cautiously opened it, and there, struggling to get out, was a huge coconut crab. Double quick, I slammed the drawer shut (coconut crabs have powerful claws for crushing the hard shells of the coconuts they feed on). The midwives laughed, telling us the crabs were delicious to eat, and I had to join them, thankful for some comic relief from our situation!

Meanwhile the storm was still raging, and we were stuck in the middle of the Pacific Ocean, with an engine that wasn't working, no radio, no life jackets and a woman in labour. Our wee boat was like a cork being tossed around in a whirlpool. Mary and I were beginning to feel sea-sick and extremely anxious. We knew there were no search and rescue facilities and the chances of us making it to Santo weren't looking good. Making it back to our families looked even less likely. We'd been praying ever since we left our island and as the storm intensified, so did our prayers. I found myself identifying with Jesus' disciples in the boat during the storm on the Sea of Galilee in new and meaningful way! Our nightmare continued.

While we waited, the men continued making efforts to get the engine going. Suddenly, we heard a strange noise coming from the boat's engine room – smoke began to pour out and we heard the noise of the engine. The boat crew were delighted, and so were all of us. Feeling much more hopeful, we slowly headed to our destination. By this time, the wind and waves were dying down, dawn was breaking, and we could see the island of Santo in the distance. We had been delivered from danger.

However, our poor patient's contractions were getting stronger and we realised she needed to be delivered, too. She wanted to push! We knew there was no stopping things at that point. After several strong pushes, a head appeared, and a baby boy was safely delivered. We were thrilled and grateful to God that we had a healthy baby, a healthy mother, and our boat was going to make it to the island.

When we docked at Santo we walked from the wharf to the hospital and arranged for a vehicle to collect mother and baby. It was now Sunday morning, a day of rest for everyone including us. Early Monday morning we headed back to Ambae with mother and baby. It was a huge relief to be safely back on dry land. Mary and I soon completed our time in the New Hebrides and headed home to New Zealand, ready to begin our midwifery training.

This time spent in the New Hebrides was my first experience of being a missionary nurse. Although I didn't know it then, this was just the beginning of my twenty-one-year-long journey as a nurse, midwife and aid worker. It was a realistic introduction to the uncertainty, challenge and personal growth that lay ahead.

6. The Diameters of the Pelvis

I commenced my midwifery training in May 1974, where I opted to live in the nurses' home so that I could concentrate on my studies. My classmates were a great group of girls and we had a lot of fun together, trying to learn such things as the diameters of the pelvis, along with other important anatomical facts. The St Helen's staff were very approachable and willing to share their knowledge, and I began my time there happily.

Unfortunately, an embarrassing incident occurred when we toured the hospital on our first day as student midwives; we'd nearly completed our tour of the wards and labour rooms which surrounded the delivery theatre, when I fainted. Everything went blank and I woke up in a hospital bed, to the sound of, 'Who do we have here?' being asked by the on-duty consultant on his rounds. 'This is one of our new students. She has just fainted,' replied the ward sister.' 'Not a good start, Nurse,' said the consultant, smiling as he walked out. I wanted to disappear into the mattress. Luckily, it was the only time I've fainted during my whole nursing career, despite traumatic situations in hospitals and clinics around the world. I'm glad I got that over with then!

Although I loved the practical aspects of our midwifery training, and gained so much experience, I struggled with some of the theory, and this was obvious to some of my instructors. One day, a tutor called me into her office. 'Nurse Walker,' she said impatiently. 'You'll never make a midwife unless you know the diameters of the pelvis. Every waking moment you need to learn this,' she said, thrusting a plastic pelvis at me, 'otherwise you won't make it,' and stormed out. She was so convinced of this, that I spent quite a bit of time worrying that she was right. But, having delivered hundreds of babies all around the world in the years that followed, I can honestly say that I never did learn those diameters. Years later, sitting on the floor at night in a tiny hut made of plastic sheeting and pieces of wood in a Somalian refugee camp housing more than 80,000 people, knowing the diameters of the pelvis just wasn't important. At the time, I was more concerned about safely delivering the young woman before me, who was suffering birthing difficulties due to circumcision scarring. I wish I could tell every young student that their training is important, but that being able to adapt to whatever life throws at them and putting the knowledge they have to practical use is what will make the difference.

7. Friendships

The friendships we make during our student years are as valuable as the skills and knowledge we gain. I'm grateful to God for all the special friends I made at St Helen's. Heather Sims continues to be a close friend and it was a joy to welcome her to Pakistan and Zambia when she visited me years later. I enjoyed showing her the sights and the hospitals where I worked, and she was even able to deliver several babies during her visits. Heather has also been a faithful prayer support partner in my life. Back in the 1970s, we had many conversations during the weekly checks of the operating theatre at St Helen's. The words she shared with me all those years ago have been important in my life and have often come to mind when I've been in challenging situations, 'Barbara, your times are in God's hands.'

At different times during my nursing and midwifery training years, there were special young men who also provided me with friendship, support and fun. I struggled with the tension between staying in New Zealand, settling down and getting married, as many of my friends were doing, or following the path I believed God was calling me on. I chose the latter, and these relationships ended. I was pleased when these young men eventually married and settled in New Zealand, following the paths that were meant for them, while I followed mine.

The early 1970s was an exciting time to be a young adult Christian living in Auckland. Many of my friends attended the popular Valley Road Baptist Church there, so I left the Anglican church I was attending and joined them. The leader of the church, Pastor Dave, had a major impact on many people's lives and as a result of his ministry, many young people went off to various Bible Colleges around New Zealand and Australia, me included. Valley Road Baptist Church had several senior mission leaders who had worked overseas in challenging places and gave me invaluable wisdom and prayer support. It was a time of spiritual training and I am grateful to all who played a part in my own spiritual formation.

In November 1974, I completed my midwifery course. This was another major achievement. I was thrilled to receive my New Zealand Registered Midwife medal. I then worked briefly as a midwife at Wairoa Hospital, a small rural hospital in Hawke's Bay. Dad was headmaster at Wairoa primary school, so I was able to spend time with my parents and young brother, but my heart wasn't in it, set as it was on becoming an Aid worker/missionary nurse; I was already planning my next move.

8. 'I Get My Directions from God, not Man…'

I still wasn't completely sure what my next step would be. Conversations with missionary nurses and mission leaders convinced me that I should look seriously at attending a Bible college before going overseas as a missionary nurse-midwife. I wanted a college that would provide both theological and practical components, and a missionary training college in Tasmania I'd heard about sounded ideal. I was accepted, and in February 1975, I headed across the Tasman Sea to Tasmania.

The college, located a few kilometres from Launceston, was to be my home for the next two years. I struggled tremendously to adjust to college life and sometimes I wondered if it was the right place for me. The rules and regulations were quite strict. By that point in my life, I had become an independent person who shared a flat and was used to having my own room and car and socialising with male friends. Sharing a dormitory with five to seven girls, many of whom would not have been my choice of roommate, was not something I was used to, and I found it very hard. The theory behind the arrangement was that on the mission field, people would be thrown together with no choice in the matter and would need to get on.

The same was true of the food we would be expected to eat; meals were served in the dining room and we were expected to eat what was put in front of us. It was all part of 'good missionary training.' For me this was prophetic: in the years that followed, I found myself being expected to eat all sorts of interesting food items such as oxen eyes, animal intestines and sheep testicles. In such situations, I prayed silently, 'Lord, I've taken it in. You keep it in!'

I did find a congenial group of like-minded friends at college. On Saturday afternoons we would 'go bush,' which involved putting on our jeans, grabbing the tea billy, tin mugs, bush tea and a bit of milk and driving to a suitable bush area where we would light a small fire to boil the billy. In places like this, we would spend our time relaxing, talking about our dreams and plans. It was important to have other people at the same stage of life to discuss the future with.

Throughout my studies, I learnt a lot about prayer, theology, church history and Bible related topics, and I learned to trust in God. One of my other favourite course topics was cross-cultural studies. I really enjoyed learning about different cultures, which laid the foundation for work that God was preparing for me in the years that lay ahead. Twice a month, visiting missionaries would stay at the college and share what life on the mission field was really like. Their stories, and faith in God, revealed to me the promise found in 1 Thessalonians 5 verse 24, 'He who calls is faithful and will equip you.' I claimed this verse as my verse and kept it close when I headed overseas.

We also learnt to equip ourselves, with practical skills that would help us to be self-sufficient in the field, including carpentry, car mechanics and plumbing. I thoroughly enjoyed these courses and these practical skills came in handy when I later helped to build feeding centres in refugee camps, and unblock toilets in our team house in Somalia. Understanding car mechanics is also useful when breaking down in the middle of the desert in Somalia, or when faced with a flat tyre on a Toyota Land Cruiser. In those days there were no roadside assistance, radio or cell phones in African countries. We simply had to solve the problem or hope someone would come along.

Life at college could be tough, and I struggled with the academic work; at times I wondered if I'd made a huge mistake. I also had some memorable interactions with the principal, Mr D. Both of us were stubborn and we clashed on several occasions. It was a challenging time. One such occasion was at the end of the second term of my first year, just as I was about to fly to New Zealand for a holiday break. The principal approached me in the dining room and said, 'Barbara, I don't think you should return to college after the break. You're not suited to this place.' Looking him in the eye, I said, 'I take my directions from God, not from man, and God has told me to be here.'

Later, when I returned from my holiday in New Zealand, the principal greeted me with these words as I climbed down from the bus: 'I told you not to return.' 'Great welcome!' I mumbled under my breath. 'God has told me to come back,' I replied, and walked into the college. Over the next few months, God slowly worked in both our lives and we began to have respect for each other. When I graduated at the end of my second year, the principal wished me well, and I was able to thank him for all I had learnt at his college. It was interesting to learn years later when I visited the college, that my intake of students in 1975 was the most challenging group the staff had had to deal with for some time. I reckon those tough years at college were part of God's wider plan, as many of us went on to serve as missionaries/Christian Aid workers in some of the world's most difficult places.

There were other challenges that presented themselves during my time in Tasmania. While I was there, I spent a great deal of time lying on a mattress on the floor, suffering from severe back problems. These occurred monthly, and meant I was often not able to carry out normal duties. I was given light duties and became the main flower arranger. My floral arrangements weren't your normal ones, but they showed flair and creativity and I was often asked to do large flower arrangements for college events. But the pain persisted, and eventually a doctor prescribed tests, x-rays, and medication. I was having trouble coping with this, not really understanding what was going on, and it got me down at times. Years later, when I was working at Bannu Hospital in Pakistan, I went for more tests and a likely diagnosis was made, but at the time, it made a normal life quite hard. I learned to live with it, and this resilience would also serve me well in later years.

Towards the end of my time there, when I was starting to wonder what would be next, a New Zealand nurse called Annette who worked in the Chacco Region of Argentina, came and shared with us stories about the medical work which she was carrying out in this region. She was looking for someone to join her. The work she was engaged in sounded both exciting and challenging, and as she shared her story with us, I began to wonder if that may be where God wanted me to go.

9. Mission, Marriage and Me: A Time to Reflect

After Annette's talk, I spent some time speaking with her, asking questions about the possibilities for me in her mission, and she encouraged me to continue to pray, while also giving me the contact address of the mission she was working with, which had its headquarters in Sydney. The organisation put me on their mailing list and kept me in their prayers. Some months later, while I was staying with friends in Sydney during the college holidays, I met the person in charge of the mission and was invited to attend their mission weekend in the Blue Mountains. This gave me an opportunity to meet mission workers, supporters and other potential recruits. A young man called Steve, (not his real name), and I had stimulating conversations about mission work, the personal cost involved and how to discern God's call for our lives. Steve lived in Sydney and we decided to stay in touch by writing letters and speaking on the phone. During this time, the mission society offered me a position in Argentina as a nurse-midwife and asked Steve and me about our future. I returned to Sydney in the following college holidays and spent time with Steve. We both began to wonder if God was calling us to the mission field as a married couple. Things moved along fast, and one evening Steve asked me to become his wife. I said yes, and we got engaged there and then. I rang my parents, who were somewhat surprised but congratulated us. Friends in Sydney arranged an engagement party to congratulate us both.

The next day I flew back to Tasmania and told my college friends I'd got engaged. 'Who to?' they asked, as I hadn't mentioned Steve to anyone. A few weeks later he came to college and met my friends. Afterwards, they shared their thoughts with me; they had serious concerns about my choice, felt we were not suited and were praying for me. As time went by, I began to have trouble sleeping at night and started to lose weight. I took some time out from college and went and stayed with friends who lived near a lovely beach. I walked on the beach for hours, pleading with God to show me if I was doing the right thing or had made a mistake. Although Steve was sure of our relationship, I was having serious doubts. One night he rang to tell me he was going to appear before the mission board. If this went well, they would look at interviewing us as a potential couple.

The night before his interview I lay awake, tossing and turning and continued praying the day of the interview. Later that day, I received a phone call from Steve. The board had turned him down. They didn't have any suitable work for him in the area where they wanted to place me. I expressed my sadness and told him I needed time to digest the news. From a simply human perspective, I longed to get married, but my heart was saying, 'Barbara, no!' God had called me to the mission field, of that

I was sure. More sleepless nights ensued. Should I go to Argentina or stay behind and marry Steve?

This was a decision I had to make with God alone, a tough decision, but I knew my call was to be a missionary nurse-midwife. Slowly, God revealed His plans for me.

I flew to Sydney and Steve came around to the house where I was staying with a girlfriend. It was there that I told Steve I couldn't marry him and that my call was to the mission field. If that meant I was to go alone, then that was what I needed to do. I wanted to honour the commitment I had made to God many years earlier at the camp. We both shed tears as we talked about my decision. Steve was very upset, as was I about the decision I had made, but deep down it was the right decision for us. We sat for a while in silence and prayed together before saying our goodbyes. Our paths have never crossed again. A few days later I contacted the mission board and announced my withdrawal from missionary service in Argentina, explaining that I needed time to come to terms with my broken engagement. I had complete trust in God, but I still yearned to know what God wanted of me and where He would lead me next.

With these questions burning in my head, I returned to college and graduated at the end of the year. During those months I thought long and hard about the decision I'd made. It was painful and hard, but I had no regrets. In 1977, I spent eight months working part-time as a parish sister for the Tasmanian Anglican Church and worked part-time as a district nurse for the local hospital. Working three days a week for the church, and three days as a district nurse, I got to know many people as patients or parishioners. They ranged from wealthy owners of sheep stations to retired people, coal miners, shop keepers, hospital staff and the community at large who lived in the three towns of St Marys, Fingal and Avoca, and outlying small villages. I enjoyed putting into practice the skills I had learnt at college and keeping my hand in with my practical district nursing. I lived in a small cottage beside the Tasman Sea, and I loved lying in bed at night listening to the sea pounding on the rocks. College friends came to stay during the holidays. It was a lovely place and gave me time to continue to think and pray about the mission field.

Later that year, I headed to England with a group of friends to do our 'big OE' (overseas experience), for a couple of months. We hired a campervan and travelled around Scotland and the north of England, explored the

Scottish Highlands and enjoyed wonderful hospitality from people living in remote areas. My friend Mary and I then joined a camping bus tour of Europe. We 'did' Europe in six weeks, visiting countries and key tourist attractions on a whirlwind tour. After the tour, I headed home to New Zealand and got a job as a midwife at St Helen's Hospital in Auckland.

Having completed my nursing, midwifery and Bible College training, it was time; I began talking to the pastor and elders of the Valley Road Baptist church regarding my call to the mission field.

10. 'You Won't Ever Make it!'

A missionary society based in Auckland was looking for midwives, for a large mission hospital in Thailand. Valley Road Baptist Church already had strong links at the place, through one of their missionary doctors and his family stationed there. After talking with the elders and the pastor, and spending time in prayer I wrote to the Missionary Society and asked them to send application papers. I received them, filled them in and sent them back.

In reply, the mission society asked me to complete several language tests, which would be undertaken both at their mission headquarters and at Auckland University. I completed these. The results were not good.

There was a big question mark over my ability to learn the Thai language. The mission board asked me to come for an interview. So, one evening, I drove into Auckland city, with my neck in a support collar, having had a car accident and suffered a whiplash injury a few days beforehand. A group of important Christian leaders were gathered around a large table. I was asked a series of questions and then the board chair said to me, 'Would you like to leave the room? We will call you back in soon.'

I duly left the room and waited to hear their decision.

After some time I was called back and the chair of the mission said to me, 'Barbara, thank you for completing our application process, sitting our languages tests and coming to see us tonight,' He continued, 'We have considered your application and feel it would be too hard for you to work in Thailand. The language is hard to learn, and we feel it would put too much pressure on you and your colleagues. We feel it would be better for you to stay in New Zealand and continue to support missionaries with your prayers and support.'

Those words still ring in my ears today. I was stunned beyond belief. My disappointment swallowed me up. A few words of encouragement were spoken, then I turned to the chair, and said politely, while holding back tears, 'Thank you for your comments, but God has called me, and I will go to the mission field,' and left the room.

I sat in my car wondering if I had got God's call on my life wrong. Had the six years of nursing and midwifery training and Bible college study been in vain? Did I get it all wrong? How did I get it so wrong?

Deeply distressed, I drove home and received wonderful support from my flatmates who were as shocked as I was. Over the next few days I went through an emotional rollercoaster, crying, thinking, questioning. I continued working at St Helen's while wondering what the future held. It wasn't an easy time.

11. One Door Closes, and Another Opens Wide

Ten days later, as I was driving home from work, I was listening to the local radio station. During a break in the songs, the announcer said World Vision was looking for nurses and doctors willing to go to Thailand to assist with the refugee crisis which was unfolding on the Thailand-Cambodian border. Thousands of Cambodian refugees were flooding across the border into Thailand to escape the brutal regime of the leader Pol Pot and his merciless supporters. This regime had been in power for some years and stories of hundreds of thousands of people being slaughtered and the growing humanitarian crisis occurring there had finally caught the world's attention. Governments and Non-Government Organizations (aid agencies) were now responding.

As I listened, I wondered if maybe this was what God had in His plans for me. I drove home, but I kept thinking about this call overnight, praying and hardly sleeping. The next day I rang the World Vision office in Auckland, explained who I was, and they arranged an appointment for me to come and see them. I went to the office where they interviewed me along with some other nurses, midwives and doctors. In the end, several us were chosen to go.

A few weeks earlier, one door had closed but now another door had opened, and I would soon be on my way. This was to be the beginning of my nursing and midwifery journey which would last nearly 21 years in many countries all over the world. My parents were wonderfully supportive of my going and drove up from their home to see me fly out to Thailand along with other members of the first New Zealand World Vision medical team. My parents knew this was something I had always felt called to do and they gave me their blessing, if a little apprehensively. With the blessing of my church, the prayer support of friends, and the somewhat concerned support of my parents, I headed off. I was on my way: God's call on my life given to me so many years ago was finally being fulfilled.

12. Sakeo One Refugee Camp, Thailand, 1979: Baptism of Fire

Between 1975 and 1979, an estimated 1.5 to 3 million Cambodians were killed in an horrific genocide under Pol Pot's dictatorship. The exact number will never be known. Pol Pot, the ruler of Cambodia, led his Khmer Rouge followers in a four-year journey of killings and torture in a plan to turn Cambodia into a Socialist, agrarian republic founded on Marxist-Leninist-Maoist policies. Anyone who opposed this regime risked their lives. City dwellers were forced into labour camps in the countryside, where mass executions, forced labour, physical abuse, disease and malnutrition eliminated a quarter of the population.

During my time working in the camps, several of our Cambodian staff shared their horrific stories with me and other World Vision staff, including their own personal stories of what happened to them and members of their families. They shared how Pol Pot's soldiers would come into cities, towns and villages, and select anyone, including educated people, doctors, pastors, women, men, children and young people, basically any one they chose, and those people were slaughtered. Our Cambodian staff shared with us stories of family members who were forced to dig graves and then kill their family members, before they too were killed by Pol Pot's soldiers. Those who showed any opposition to the regime were executed in the Killing Fields and thrown into mass graves. The genocide ended in 1979 when the Vietnamese invaded Cambodia and defeated the Khmer Rouge regime. Pol Pot, along with some of his soldiers, headed for the Thailand border, near to where I would later be working.

Those first days in Thailand were a baptism of fire, a dramatic introduction to the plight of Cambodian refugees, their trauma, and the enormity of human suffering. The Thai government had provided the land for the refugee camps to be built on, and aid agencies from around the world arrived to help. World Vision New Zealand was amongst several relief agencies which were assigned to assist in the Sakeo One refugee camp.

Although we'd been told about the conditions at Sakeo One, nothing could have prepared us for the sight. As we drove through the gates of the camp, we saw thousands of flimsy bamboo huts covered in United Nations High Commission for Refugees standard green plastic sheeting. We climbed out of the van and walked around the camp. Hundreds of displaced people were squatting in a large area not far from their hastily built huts, just staring at us. Their faces were expressionless. No one spoke. Their humanity had been grimly suppressed under Pol Pot's regime where any form of emotion was punishable by torture. Many of these refugees had witnessed the most awful atrocities, including the execution of family members. They were like zombies. Everyone wore black. It was exceptionally eerie. A male member of our team kicked a football towards a group of children. It was an invitation to play. At first the children looked and did nothing, and then slowly, hesitantly, they began to respond.

Afterwards, we were taken on a tour of the hastily constructed bamboo hospital which was shrouded in more of the plastic sheeting. I'd never seen anything like it. I'd come straight from the modern St Helen's Hospital in Auckland, New Zealand, to a hastily built bamboo structure which housed hundreds of critically ill, traumatised Cambodian refugees.

The hospital consisted of wards run by different aid agencies from countries all over the world who were responding to this humanitarian disaster. The World Vision ward was a large, unbelievably crowded area filled with bamboo slat beds, in which patients lay, only a few feet apart. There were no mattresses, sheets or blankets. Most of the patients in this ward were seriously ill with cerebral malaria, and suffering from feverish deliriums, causing many of them to fit. My friend Jo and I volunteered to go on duty that night – how we longed to relieve this incredible suffering! We reported for duty in our cotton trousers and tops which we had brought from home, uniforms not being important in these surroundings.

After being given a few basic instructions, we were thrown in the deep end, as lead nurses in charge of the ward for the night. A nurse who'd just arrived a few weeks earlier gave us a crash course in inserting intravenous drips into patients' arms. We worked at a frenetic pace, inserting drips to administer the Valium and quinine intravenously to those who had been diagnosed as having cerebral malaria. More patients kept arriving throughout the night from the nearby emergency tent, which was run by a highly competent Israeli medical team, with cerebral malaria being the most common diagnosis, along with some people with pneumonia.

The helpers assigned to Jo and me during that night, and in many to follow in Sakeo One, were mostly former Pol Pot Khmer Rouge girl soldiers who knew no English but had been assigned to the ward by the camp authorities. To this day I don't know why these girls were assigned to help, nor do I know if they had had any basic first aid training; it was politically wise in a situation like that to accept what the authorities said and not ask too many questions.

Our first night in Sakeo One was a tough one. Many patients died from complications of cerebral malaria. Their bodies were carried away by the girl soldiers to be cremated in the camp's rudimentary incinerator. When morning came, we were absolutely shattered. As we travelled back to our team house, I wondered if I'd got my guidance wrong. Did I have the stamina and strength to continue to work in such tough conditions? But after the first few days, I knew I could carry on with God's help.

Our medical team lived in basic wooden houses which World Vision had rented from local villagers. Local Thai people were employed to cook our meals, and the locally employed World Vision driver drove us to and from the bamboo hospital. The village was poor; many skinny scrawny dogs which could be carrying rabies or worms, roamed freely; there was no SPCA to call, so they just wandered around looking for food and fighting amongst themselves. They were just one of many strange things (and potential dangers) we would have to become accustomed to, and we had to admire the animals' ability to adapt.

Sometimes the dangers came from unexpected places. One day I was on duty and heard that one of our nurses had been shot in one of our team houses. Information slowly filtered through. It was her day off and she had been sitting up in bed, when a Thai man in the house next door had pulled the trigger on the gun, he was cleaning, not realising it was loaded. The bullet shot through the wall, entered one side of the nurse's mouth and exited the other. If she'd been sitting a little higher, she would have been killed. Hurrying to her house, a medical team assessed the situation, identified one of our team members with the same blood group and did a person-to-person blood transfusion. The injured nurse was transported to Bangkok for immediate medical assistance and then flown home to America for reconstructive surgery.

Many years later, I was at a conference in Pakistan and met a fascinating American woman. We talked about places we'd worked in and she told me she'd been shot while working in a refugee camp in Thailand. I realised she was the nurse who'd been shot at Sakeo One! Joan told me more of her story and what had happened to her when she got back to America after she had been shot. She was now fully recovered and only had a very small scar on her face. Meeting her after all those years was truly a God moment, and testament to the resilience of others who had been called to serve in these places.

As news about the tragically unfolding humanitarian situation reached the rest of the world, telex messages and offers of aid began pouring in. A group of American mothers who were living in America even contacted the American Embassy in Bangkok, volunteering to come and breast-feed orphans. We at World Vision were asked if we would like to accept this very generous offer but after talking with the team, we thanked them for their concern and declined their offer. They were just one group who was responding to the horrific news that had started to spread around the world.

13. Bamboo Hospitals in a Bamboo City

After we had been a few weeks at Sakeo One, World Vision asked if some of us would be willing to help establish a new camp at Khao I Dang nearer the Cambodian border. I accepted this offer without hesitation, as the camp in Sakeo One was well staffed, and I was ready to use my skills elsewhere. Seven of us drove from Sakeo One to a place nearer to the Cambodian border, passing through the town of Aranyaprathet to a small village, near where World Vision had managed to rent a couple of team houses, 20 kilometres by road from Khao I Dang.

At Khao I Dang, the Thai government had allocated a barren stretch of wasteland with no convenient water supply for the camp. The government had invited the UNHCR and multiple aid agencies to come and build a new refugee camp, which soon consisted of a large bamboo hospital (another hospital was built later), offices, and warehouses to store the tons of food which was being trucked in regularly to feed the refugees. The aid agencies also assisted the refugees with building supplies so that they could build their own huts. Khao I Dang grew quickly. At its height, it was the world's largest refugee camp, housing more than 120,000 Cambodian refugees. Water was trucked in from neighbouring towns and toilets were hastily dug. The Thai government rapidly constructed a barbed-wire fence around the huge camp, with only one entrance point. Thai armed guards were placed around the outside of the fence to prevent the refugees escaping.

We began work on the World Vision ward, helped by a team of willing Cambodians. Putting my basic carpentry training from Bible College to good use, I wielded a hammer to nail up lengths of bamboo and cut and installed sheets of plastic for the walls. Labouring in the hot, humid, dusty conditions was incredibly hard work, but an immense structure of bamboo poles began to take shape. Building supplies were trucked in daily and the frame was quickly encased in thick UNHCR plastic sheeting. In our ward, we covered the floors with more plastic sheeting and built a modified nurses' station from which we could observe everyone in the ward, before placing dozens of bamboo beds each side of the aisle. Patients would later lie on these bamboo beds, some with pieces of material to lie on and others with lightweight blankets. Some patients would have nothing. Everything was pitifully basic.

Soon after construction was finished, hundreds of new refugees began to arrive in buses each day from the border and those who had been injured arrived in the back of large trucks. These people often arrived in critical condition, after stepping on land mines, being injured from gun fire, becoming critically ill from cerebral malaria or severely dehydrated from diarrhoea and vomiting. Sadly, many of the sick and injured died in the trucks, or soon after arriving at camp.

Triage teams assessed the wounded, sorting out those needing urgent help. These patients were sent to the Emergency Ward run by a dedicated team of German surgeons, nurses and technicians working under unbelievably difficult circumstances, with few drugs or surgical aids. Everyone rejoiced one morning when a complete operating theatre was flown in from Germany to Bangkok and then trucked to the camp. The German medical team quickly got the operating theatre tents assembled and were able to carry out life-saving operations.

Most of our patients were adults with surgical and medical conditions who arrived at our ward having had surgery for broken limbs, or basic repairs to shattered legs resulting from land mines. Some also came with gunshot wounds or were suffering from cerebral malaria, pneumonias, unknown fevers, abscesses, severe dehydration and severe abdominal pains caused by dysentery. We also had some children in our ward, who sadly were suffering from similar conditions. We had patients who were so traumatized by what they had seen and personally experienced that they just sat or lay on their bamboo beds and refused to eat or talk.

The once empty fields at Khao I Dang very soon became a bustling city with two bamboo hospitals caring for over 1,500 patients at the height of the crisis. There were over a hundred doctors, nurses, midwives and other aid workers from around the world working in the camp in those early days. Despite these numbers, we were chronically short-staffed, due to the extreme needs of the patients, so our wonderful Kiwi doctor, Robin Briant, taught the nurses how to diagnose, giving us basic training in identifying the most common health problems: malaria, pneumonia, skin infections and post-surgical cases. She taught us how to listen to chest sounds using a stethoscope and how to palpate abdomens. There was a basic laboratory in the camp that could process many kinds of blood tests; this laboratory was always very busy and grew as more equipment and people arrived to help. Each nurse was assigned a certain number of patients with Dr Robin on hand to answer questions and help. It was a huge step up and a steep learning curve for a New Zealand country girl!

I learnt so much there and gained practical skills and experience which proved invaluable for working overseas in disaster situations. I also learnt about myself, my feelings, the need to trust God's leading, and to pace myself when working in stressful environments. From my patients, I learnt the incredible power of the human spirit to overcome adversity, seeing how they were so grateful simply to be alive and safe.

Many of the patients also spoke of their amazing trust in God, stories which were translated by the Cambodian interpreters we relied on to communicate with our patients; talented young people who had managed to escape from Pol Pot's tyrannical regime and were now employed by World Vision. My interpreter was a young man called Danny who had been a disc jockey on Radio Phnom Penh years earlier, before he had fled to Thailand. He had heard about the plight of his people who were streaming into the camps and came to Khao I Dang wanting to help his sick compatriots by translating for them. The horror of what these young interpreters had witnessed under Pol Pot's rule began to emerge as they felt safe to confide in us. They told tragic stories of witnessing family members being killed, hacked to death, often in front of them, and other unimaginable horrors, many of which it is not my place to tell. They spoke of their struggle to find food and medical care when they were ill, and of living in an environment of abject fear.

Many also spoke of their faith in God and of wonderful answers to prayer: some were in their twenties but had the faith of people much older and more experienced; they were wise elders in the Christian faith, and in comparison, I felt I was still in kindergarten. One day, during my first few days in Khao I Dang, a Cambodian pastor asked if he could do a regular Bible study in our ward and pray with the patients. Many patients' lives, and the lives of their families who were with them, were touched through these studies and prayer. The pastor shared with us that God had spoken to him and encouraged him to lead his congregation from Batumbong in Cambodia through the Killing Fields and across the border to safety into Khao I Dang. This was a very dangerous thing to do, as Pol Pot's regime was targeting Christians and hundreds had been killed.

As Cambodian Christians shared the word of God with their fellow Cambodians, the Spirit of God began to move through Khao I Dang. For the first time, many Cambodian refugees in this camp heard about God's love for them and committed their lives to Jesus Christ. This message of salvation came from their own people; Cambodian Christians who had endured those terrible years and knew the reality of God's power and love. Hundreds of refugees began to attend the Cambodian church services, which were run by the refugee pastors, and as the weeks went by, more and more refugees attended. At times, we struggled to get Cambodian staff to help at the hospital because they wanted to attend Bible studies and prayer meetings. These Cambodian Christians were praying not only for their own people, but also for the hundreds of foreign aid workers who were coming to assist in this humanitarian crisis; their generosity moved us all.

One Sunday morning, I attended a memorable open-air church service with hundreds of refugees. We sat on the ground and listened to the Cambodians singing their hymns. This was truly amazing, as for years under Pol Pot's rule anything remotely Christian was not allowed and anyone who broke this rule was killed or severely tortured. A song with words like the popular hymn 'All to Jesus I Surrender,' touched me deeply. These people had truly surrendered all and many of their families and friends had been killed. Whenever I hear that song, I am transported back to that church service. The persecuted church has much to teach Western Christians, but we are often too busy to listen.

I had my own revelations during my time at Khao I Dang; at one point, I had the opportunity to travel to a hospital where I had applied to work some months earlier with the New Zealand mission organisation that had turned me down. I met some extremely dedicated people at the hospital and yet, as I was leaving to head back to camp, I knew deep down this wasn't the place for me. It had been hard to bear when that door closed some months earlier, but God now had me in the place where He wanted me. This strengthened my faith in Him.

These spiritual encounters lifted us up, but the physical reality of our day-to-day life kept us grounded. Living in primitive conditions took its toll, and every team member eventually succumbed to diarrhoea and chest infections. I soon became ill, with symptoms of aching bones, fever, severe eye pain, headaches and a rash. Just before Christmas 1979, I was driven to the Bangkok Nursing Home Hospital, a very good hospital in Thailand's capital city. Blood tests revealed that I had contracted dengue fever, a disease spread by mosquitoes. The symptoms are high fevers, a rash, muscle and joint pains and severe headaches. In severe cases there can be serious bleeding and shock which can be life threatening. There is no treatment for this disease, apart from pain relief, a cream for the itchy rash, Valium and a lot of rest. I spent a lot of time sleeping; working all hours in the camp hospital had been exceptionally demanding and I was exhausted.

The nursing home was set in beautiful gardens, and the British Matron called in regularly to check on me. It was an ideal place to rest and after five days I began to recover. The Christmas day menu included turkey and all the trimmings, but sadly the dengue fever limited my appetite. When I was discharged, the doctor instructed me to have two weeks off to fully recover, before heading back to the camp. The question was where to recover? I had a sudden brainwave.

14. Another Happy Coincidence

My mother's sister June Inder and her husband Peter were at Recsan University in Penang, Malaysia, where Peter was teaching, and I decided that I should go there. Coincidentally, I'd heard that my parents and younger brother Philip happened to be holidaying there at the time. Although I had my uncle and aunt's address, I didn't have their phone number. So, I flew to Penang airport, hired a taxi, and told the driver to drop me at my uncle's house.

A house guard answered the door and I asked to see Uncle Peter. My uncle was astonished to see me standing on his doorstep, but quickly invited me inside. I followed him into the kitchen and there, sitting at the table, were my Dad, my brother and my aunt. They were even more surprised to see me. Giving me a hug and a cold drink, Dad asked, 'What are you doing here? Who told you?' 'Told me what?' I asked. 'Your Mum is upstairs. She's had a heart attack and is on strict bed rest.'

Shocked, I dropped my bag and sank into a chair.

'No-one told me,' I managed, 'I've been in hospital in Bangkok with dengue fever. I'm not allowed back to work for two weeks and so I thought I'd come here; I didn't have your phone number so here I am.' 'Its lovely to see you,' they all said.

'I'll tell your mother you're here,' said Dad. 'She'll get a huge surprise.'

I had a cold drink while I waited for Dad to come downstairs.

'Mum wants to see you,' said Dad, so I slowly climbed the stairs and entered Mum's bedroom. She gave me a big hug and told me what had happened. She'd had a heart attack while travelling in Penang. 'Did your father call you and tell you to come?' she enquired. 'No, I'm on sick leave,' I explained. 'Fortunately, dengue fever isn't contagious!'

I spent a pleasant two weeks with my relatives, sleeping, eating and catching up on family news. The local GP checked on Mum daily and felt she would get more rest at Uncle Peter's place than in a busy hospital ward. Also, the cost of a coronary care unit in Penang was outside my parent's insurance budget. Mum and I slowly recovered and enjoyed the chance to catch up properly. After our joint recuperation, she was checked out by a cardiologist in Singapore before flying back to New Zealand and I returned to camp two weeks later.

15. Back to the Largest Bamboo City in the World

On my return to Khao I Dang, I discovered that many of my colleagues had also caught dengue fever. Depression can be a serious side effect of this, and sadly, one team member developed this condition and was repatriated. It was a hard time for all of us, as we struggled to cope with the ongoing challenges of very sick refugees arriving daily, the very hot humid weather, and continual episodes of stomach upsets. It really was down to just taking one day at a time.

As a midwife, I was called on by Cambodian traditional birth attendants to help when they ran into difficulties when they were delivering babies. I discovered that Cambodians have some interesting post-delivery customs. After the baby has been delivered, mother and baby lie on a bamboo slat bed with a coal-filled metal oven placed underneath. It is the husband's job to keep the fire going. This practice is believed to help reduce the mother's post-delivery bleeding. We felt somewhat dubious about this custom as Cambodia, like Thailand, is hot all year round; this practice had to be monitored to ensure mothers and babies didn't suffer dehydration. We encouraged the mother to drink plenty of water and to feed her baby regularly. This was part of their cultural practices and something which we observed frequently. We were aware that, working cross-culturally, people must be very sensitive to the customs and practices of other cultures and beliefs.

We did have the occasional break. During my time in Khao I Dang, a few of us New Zealand World Vision workers were invited to stay at the New Zealand Embassy in Bangkok. This invitation from the New Zealand ambassador to Thailand, Richard Taylor, and his wife, came about following a visit Mr Taylor had made to the camp hospital.

We were invited to come to Bangkok as their guests for Waitangi Day celebrations, and we duly travelled down by train. At the event, a Māori concert group provided wonderful entertainment while we mingled with guests. We stayed at the embassy and the ambassador's chauffeur drove us around the sights of Bangkok. It was a lovely break from the challenges and pressures of Khao I Dang. Following the ambassador's visit to the camp, he got word back to our families in New Zealand, informing them we were well and doing a wonderful job. This meant a lot to my parents.

After this little reprieve, I returned to Khao I Dang for a few more months before my contract expired in June 1980. World Vision was offering longer contracts for the new nurses and doctors arriving, but I was ready to move on.

16. The Boat People: Desperation, Danger and Hope

When my contract in Thailand ended, I decided to help in another humanitarian crisis unfolding not far away in another South-East Asian country. North Vietnam had invaded South Vietnam in 1975, and thousands of South Vietnamese were fleeing from the turmoil and conflict out into the South China Sea on flimsy, overcrowded fishing boats. Desperate to escape, thousands of these people were paying outrageous sums of money to unscrupulous fishing boat owners in the hope of reaching places like Indonesia, or even far-away Australia. They were prepared to risk their lives to find a new homeland and peace.

As a westerner, I stand in awe of these people who chose to take this enormous risk. Having paid the money, mothers, fathers, children, young people and whole families joined other desperate individuals and streamed onto small boats to sail into the unknown. Many of these boats were unseaworthy and certainly not built for venturing into the turbulent waters of the South China Sea. The possibility of these people being killed by pirates or drowning in storms was extremely high, but the risks of staying in their country and being killed were higher. What a choice they had to make. Although an estimated 300,000 boat people had died, thousands were still escaping this way or drifting on the ocean in 'floating coffins.' If they did reach a foreign shore, they were never sure whether that country would take them in. International law required these boat people to be taken to the nearest port. Countries like Indonesia opened their doors to the boat people, while other countries like Malaysia and Singapore closed theirs.

To try to relieve this humanitarian crisis, World Vision purchased a large coastal freighter and christened it *Seasweep*, as it was the first international rescue ship 'sweeping the sea' to locate the boat people and provide food and medical care to any they found. I understood from the World Vision staff based in Singapore that it had taken the captain and crew members months attempting to get the ship registered in ten different countries, before finally succeeding in Honduras. President of World Vision International, Stanley Mooneyham, decided in mid-1979 that World Vision would assist the boat people, despite opposition from governments in the area. Mooneyham was very concerned that *Seasweep* wouldn't be able to rescue all the boat people because of the numbers attempting escape, and worried which country would accept them. The focus of operation Seasweep in those early days was to support the people to stay on their boats, rather than taking them onboard the *Seasweep* herself.

When I joined *Seasweep* in June 1980, I found it was a well-organized operation. I quickly became part of a small international medical team of eight, two of whom had just completed a six-week contract and were staying on. Our team included two doctors, four nurses and two technical people who were able to ensure that all the equipment we needed was working. They were helped by an Indonesian crew, who assisted us in practical ways as needed. As new recruits, we were given a tour of the ship and I, being a nurse, was particularly interested in seeing what medical supplies were on board. I was delighted to find a basic medical clinic with first aid equipment – bandages, disinfectants, antibiotics and other medicines, vaccinations and IV drips. The mission of *Seasweep* at that time was to rescue the people in the refugee boats and take them to holding camps which had been set up in Indonesia.

On the day of our departure, I received sad news via a telegram; my Wellington grandmother had died. Nana Ruby, my father's mother, was a special, colourful woman, and a gifted milliner. She was a staunch member of the Labour Party and the National Council of Women and not afraid of speaking up on issues, a quality I admired in her and inherited. I knew that Nana Ruby would want me to continue the work

I was doing, and so I said my private farewells, and decided to continue with this new challenge.

In June 1980, we sailed from the safety of Singapore Harbour and headed into the open sea where we would spend the next six weeks searching for boat people. We were embarking on a difficult and dangerous mission: no-one knew what lay ahead. It was a suspenseful time, but I felt at peace, knowing that God was with us. We had been warned about the severe storms which can arise very suddenly in the area, as well as the constant threat of pirates. Every morning we had a short team meeting, where the day was planned as far as it could be, and then we had a time of prayer. The captain and crew members continuously scanned the horizon with binoculars, searching for boat people.

During my first week on *Seasweep* we intercepted the first vessel, a small, dangerously overloaded boat pitching and tossing in the rolling ocean. On board we found 45 people huddled on the deck, underneath tarpaulins. 'We've come to help you,' the captain shouted through a megaphone. 'We are going to draw alongside.' Members of our crew lowered the steel ladder and slowly the people on the boat began to clamber up. The children were lifted to the ship first, followed by the adults, and members of the medical team held onto them tightly until their parents arrived. Over the next hour, we managed to get them all on board; they were safe. Many of the refugees were dehydrated from lack of water and food. We fed them, gave them water, and then began to see if any of them had any other health concerns. We helped the boat people down another ladder into the bowels of the ship, where we had stores of clothing, food, water and blankets.

A Vietnamese man who seemed like a leader of the group said they had suffered a broken engine and mast, and Thai pirates operating in the area had stolen their valuables, food, maps, money and compasses. They were then left to drift in this huge ocean. They had managed to survive thus far on rainwater and scanty rations, risking their lives because they were so desperate to get out of war-torn South Vietnam.

Few spoke English, but in situations like that, the language of love transcends words. Many smiled and hugged us, weeping with gratitude, and others thanked us in broken English. Tears streamed down our faces as we ministered to each other. The joy cannot be expressed in words. Memories of that day will be forever etched on my mind. They told harrowing stories of violent storms and of being attacked and robbed by pirates. Sorrowfully, they spoke of the many boats that had sunk and the people who had drowned. To this day, no one knows exactly how many people fled South Vietnam and how many drowned in their search for freedom.

One man, Bao, spoke excellent English. He was a Christian who had emigrated to America and lectured in animal husbandry at a university. We sat on the deck, and Bao told me he'd returned to Vietnam to gather his family to bring them to America, intending to leave Vietnam for good. During his time in South Vietnam, the political situation was becoming more unsettled and Bao decided it was time for him to get his family out of his country of birth. He had spent all his savings to pay for his wife, two children and himself to board a small fishing boat and head out to sea, along with these other desperate people. His family knew the risk of storms and pirates but had no choice, as the country was in great political turmoil. He spoke of his family's deep faith in God and how being rescued by the *Seasweep* was truly an answer to their prayers. Taking my hand and, with tears streaming down his face, he said a most heartfelt, 'Thank you.' Tears flooded my eyes and I felt humbled and privileged to have played a small part in rescuing this man and his family. Over the next few weeks we picked up more than 250 refugees.

As our ship headed towards the camps for boat people, which the Indonesian government had established on islands throughout the Indonesian archipelago, we spent time attending to the basic medical needs of those in our care, giving vaccinations and recording their personal details in readiness for the camps. The stories we heard were repeated over and over: persecution, killings, poverty, rape, desperation and a final attempt to escape by boat. At the resettlement camps, the boat people were screened and then sent on to places like Canada, Australia, the USA and New Zealand, their fates unknown, but with hope to accompany them.

Incredibly, we are still hearing stories like this today, of Middle Eastern people risking their lives on overcrowded and unseaworthy boats, in the hope of reaching safety and finding a new life. Thousands lose their lives, yet they are prepared to take the risk of fleeing rather than experiencing gruesome horrors in their war-torn countries. In 1980, when I met Bao, little did I know that three decades later, boat people – now called asylum seekers – would continue to risk their lives to find freedom, safety and a better life. Sadly, for many, the better life never comes.

17. Night Sisters, Rules, and Restrictions

When my six-week contract on *Seasweep* ended, I returned to New Zealand and secured a position as a staff nurse at Greenlane Hospital in Auckland. I was placed in a medical ward and was rostered to cover all duties, including morning, afternoon and night duty. I found transitioning to the role of nurse difficult; I'd been doing the work of a house surgeon-registrar in the refugee camps of Sakeo One and Khao I Dang in Thailand, and then on the *Seasweep*. It was an anti-climax to be back in New Zealand working as a registered nurse, but I had to get used to it. I knew it would be for a limited time and then I would be heading overseas again.

A few days after I started, I was assigned to a week of night duty on the Cardiac Ward, along with another registered nurse and an aide. During the night, we had regular visits from the Nurse Night Supervisor who seemed to delight in sneaking up behind us, to make sure that we weren't asleep; I never did sleep on the job.

Early one morning, just as dawn was breaking, the emergency bell rang. I raced to the room to find a patient had collapsed in her bed, with three startled roommates looking on. We had rehearsed emergency procedures many times during our training; while my colleague rang for help, I pulled the curtains, lowered her bed and began mouth-to-mouth resuscitation, alternating it with cardiac massage. A doctor arrived, followed by the night sister. 'Get a drip inserted!' the doctor yelled as he and the Night Sister took over providing the mouth to mouth and cardiac massage. I grabbed IV drip equipment off the emergency trolley and inserted the drip into the patient's arm. More helpers arrived, so I stood back and let more experienced people take over. Sadly, after nearly half-an-hour of concentrated effort, the patient died. The doctor stopped resuscitation, thanked us all and left with his team. The morning staff arrived, and I signed off duty and drove home to get some sleep.

But I tossed and turned in bed, thinking of the patient, her family and her three roommates. I was upset we hadn't been able to save her, even though we'd tried our best. Returning to the hospital for my next shift, I was told the Night Sister wanted to see me immediately. I knocked on her door and entered with fear and trepidation. 'Staff Nurse Walker,' she said angrily. 'Who gave you permission to insert a drip into a patient? Nurses don't do that. It's not our role.'

'The doctor asked for someone to insert a drip and I've had lots of experience with inserting drips in refugee camps,' I replied. 'So, I just did it. No one else was available at the time.' She fixed me with a steely glare. 'Staff Nurse Walker, you are not overseas now. Don't do it again!'

I thanked her and returned to the ward, realising I needed to nurse in the framework of the New Zealand Nursing Council at that time. (That was in the early 1980s, but nowadays it is routine practice for nurses to insert drips into patients – in fact, nurses insert more drips than doctors.) Back in those days in New Zealand, where the role of each health professional was separate and clearly defined, it was a huge contrast for me, having worked in the refugee camps where we had thousands of patients, few doctors and a few more nurses. There weren't such clearly defined roles; as I was clearly finding out, being back in a New Zealand hospital. If I was going to continue to work in that environment, I was going to have to relearn fast. The question running around in my mind was: 'Do I really want to nurse in New Zealand?'

Heading home to the flat where I was staying, I was still challenged, mulling over differing expectations of nurses and their roles. 'God, where does my future lie?' I prayed. That afternoon, I was awakened by a phone call from World Vision New Zealand. They said a major refugee crisis was developing in Somalia, in the Horn of Africa, and doctors, nurses, midwives and engineers were urgently required. Would I go? My spirit leapt. 'Yes!' I replied without a moment's hesitation. So, this was to be my future! Thank you, God.

The following day, I went into the New Zealand World Vision office to sign another contract with World Vision International and confirmed my availability. They said I would be flying out in one week's time. A mad scramble ensued to update my passport, obtain visas, organise suitable clothing, and pack my bags. I made an appointment to see the matron and told her about the job offer. She was very understanding and released me, wishing me all the best. I never did work at Greenlane Hospital again.

Barbara Walker

18. Heat, Dust, Little Water, and Purple Hands

In the 1970s, the country of Somalia was encountering many problems, many of which were linked to the Ogaden region, which straddles the man-made border between Somalia and Ethiopia. These skirmishes, which started in the mid 1960s, erupted into a full-on assault by Somalia on the Ogaden region in 1977. This region is an area which Somalia believes was unjustly given to Ethiopia when the British and Italians withdrew from the area in 1960. Several factors led to extreme situations, forcing inhabitants to flee. The UN announced in January 1980 that Somalia had 375,000 refugees in camps, and 650,000 in towns and villages in the area. *TIME Magazine* in June 1980 stated that the Horn of Africa, which includes Somalia, Dijbouti, Eritrea and Ethiopia, had 1.7 million refugees from unresolved conflicts. Las Dhure was a microcosm of the world's worst refugee problems, which had inundated Somali camps with up to 900,000 displaced persons, according to government figures at that time.

I was heading to Las Dhure not to comment on the politics or to criticize the cultural practices and beliefs I would soon encounter, but to assist where I could, using my nursing and midwifery skills. From my earliest days as an aid worker, we were told not to comment on the politics of the country where we were working and to always remember that we were guests in that country, which for me was very wise advice.

An unfortunate start

In July 1980, I was on my way to my next assignment with World Vision International, 12 months in Somalia, joining a medical team in Las Dhure refugee camp. Our nearest country was Djibouti. Information coming out of Somalia at the time was very limited, and I left New Zealand not really knowing what I would find when I reached it, but I was willing to go and help in any way I could. I flew from Auckland to Singapore and then on to Karachi Airport in Pakistan, where we sat waiting on the tarmac for a very long time. It transpired that the vice-president of China was joining our flight. Suddenly, the seats filled with Chinese officials in grey-black uniforms and we settled in for our onward flight. On landing in Kenya, passengers were told to remain in their seats until the Chinese entourage had disembarked. Through my cabin window, I could see red carpet being rolled out and Kenyan President Daniel arap Moi and dignitaries lining up to welcome the Chinese delegation. While these formalities took place, we sweltered on the plane for more than an hour in suffocating heat, our patience wearing thin. Eventually, we were permitted to disembark, only to endure another tedious wait at customs and immigration.

There, a towering West African man in a flowing gown and matching head-dress was waiting to meet me. Joshua, who had distinctive tribal markings on his face, was World Vision International's African relief director. Joshua drove me to the hotel where I was to stay for a few nights. A crowd had gathered outside the hotel and a red carpet was being rolled out; the Chinese vice-president was due to arrive at the hotel, too! We were ushered through a vast foyer that was resplendent with chandeliers, gold-framed paintings and huge floral arrangements. I had never seen such a magnificent place.

Although Joshua had a confirmation slip, the desk clerk could find no booking for a Barbara Walker, so I was shown to a small room by the swimming pool; it looked like a changing room to me. But it had a bed, toilet and shower, so I thought, 'This will do.' Exhausted after umpteen hours of sitting on planes and waiting for vice-presidents, I just wanted to sleep, but decided to get something to eat beforehand. I wandered around the hotel looking for some food. Everyone was running around because of the VIP's arrival, so I ordered an egg sandwich and a drink from the coffee bar.

Returning to my little room, I fell asleep. I woke hours later feeling decidedly queasy. Over the next four hours the toilet and I spent quite a lot of time together! I waited until 7.30 in the morning to ring Joshua and tell him I needed a doctor. There was a doctor's surgery some distance from the hotel, so Joshua arranged for a driver to come and take me there. We finally arrived at the doctor's surgery and I staggered up two flights of stairs, walked into the surgery and collapsed at the reception desk. I was extremely dehydrated. I was helped into the doctor's room and after a very quick examination he explained that it looked like I had a bad case of food poisoning and he would refer me to the Nairobi Private Hospital for admission and treatment. The driver then took me to the hospital, where I was admitted, given intravenous fluids and told

I would be in hospital for a few days. I didn't protest, as I felt as though I'd been hit by a truck.

Joshua visited me, and the hotel owners sent a lovely bunch of flowers, thinking I'd picked up a dose of food poisoning in their hotel, though it could have been something that I had eaten on the plane. I will never know; all I wanted to do was to get better. A few days later, I was discharged from the hospital and spent the next week in the penthouse suite on the top floor, courtesy of the hotel. I felt hugely embarrassed about having to delay my departure for Somalia; a relief nurse shouldn't get sick before she arrives on the field!

After my ten-day delay in Kenya, I finally flew to Somalia in north-east Africa, over 1,800 kilometres away from Nairobi, and on to Mogadishu, the capital of Somalia, landing at the international airport. Nothing anyone would expect to find at a country's major airport was there; no immigration or customs checks. I just wandered through and collected my bags. A fellow aid worker met me and drove me through the hot, bustling streets of the capital city to the shared team house. That night we went to dinner at a nice-looking restaurant with an impressive menu, but unfortunately most of the dishes weren't available and we ate pasta with a dribble of tomato sauce, which we washed down with a bottle of Coca Cola. Talk about a taste of things to come!

A few days later, I flew up to Hargeisa, 800 km northwest of Mogadishu on a Somalia Airlines flight. Because of the fighting between Somalia and Ethiopia over the Ogaden desert region at the time, it was too dangerous for expatriates to travel by road, so flying was the only option for us. Hargeisa was a hot, dry, dusty city with a fragile infrastructure; sometimes there was no water or electricity, but there was always dust, dust and more dust. The camp at Las Dhure was a one to two-hour drive from Hargeisa, depending on road and weather conditions. So many things about that country were at the mercy of the weather; heavy rain, which came infrequently during my time in Somalia, turned dirt roads into quagmires of mud, and dry riverbeds became raging torrents, making the tracks leading to Las Dhure virtually impassable. On the other hand, the rain was a blessing, turning the desert into a multi-coloured carpet of flowers. Sadly, the flowers only lasted a few days, but the rains were welcome relief from the heat and dust that enveloped the area most of the time.

Purple Hands

Our staff compound was made up of a collection of white tents, and I was assigned a two-person tent to share with a nutritionist. We slept on canvas stretchers, placed plastic sheeting over the dirt floor, made furniture out of cardboard medicine boxes, and used a kerosene lantern and torch at night. Our pit latrine toilet had a friendly spider living under the seat. This was a bit of a change from my penthouse suite, but it was enough.

We regularly received hundreds of refugees, who were trucked into the camp. They were seeking food, shelter, medical help and safety, leaving behind the fighting and famine which had been all around them. There was a mixture of elderly, families, orphans, young men, young women, and hundreds of children and babies. Our compound was on a slight hill above the camp spread out below us; a sea of blue and green plastic sheeting provided by the United Nations High Commission for Refugees (UNHCR.) On arrival in the camp, we gave the new refugees the UNHCR plastic sheeting and blankets. Many of the new arrivals used sticks and bits of material they had brought with them to start to construct their huts. Others used anything they could find in the camp to construct a shelter for their families. These 'eggshell' dome type huts stretched across the horizon in neat rows as far as the eye could see, housing upwards of 80,000 refugees. It was a daunting sight, especially since we only had one doctor, five nurses and a nutritionist in my early days there.

It all seemed like an impossible situation. We often saw hundreds of patients a day, but we just had to focus on the next person in front of us. The world's eyes were focussed on the Cambodian refugees in Thailand and aid agencies were sending relief support and medical staff there. Somalia was very much a poor cousin, despite the scale of its human misery. The camp continued to grow, and we continued to work long hours, struggling with the heat, the dust, the sandstorms and worst of all, the millions of flies. These large flies were everywhere, crawling over our skin, up our noses, around our eyes, constantly buzzing. They would fly into our mouths and get caught in our throats; I often had coughing fits because of flies. I would be talking to someone and a fly would fly into my mouth and buzz around! I lost count of how many flies I swallowed. Often, the flies were so bad we had to sit under a mosquito net to eat meals in the corrugated iron shed in our compound, where we had a table and a few chairs. But we knew, and acknowledged each day, that this inconvenience was only that; we just had to look around us to find real suffering.

It was the children that really got to us. As we wandered around the camp, many of them would crowd around, wanting to touch us, to touch our faces. Some of the children were happy and laughed like children all around the world. Many had forgotten how to smile; their eyes showed their pain and their silent cry for help. Those who couldn't run around just lay in the shelters, waiting to die. The flies came and crawled all over the small bodies as they lay in the stinking hot huts. The smell from the vomit and faeces was just awful. Death visited frequently in those early days. Some days there were many more deaths than births. As I looked into the faces of these little children, I sometimes wondered where God was.

Sadness, tragedy and despair were all around, but despite the daily heartache, life continued in this city of plastic sheeting and cardboard boxes, dust and flies. We continued to do our best. Still, I often felt utterly helpless and useless: there were so many of them and so few of us. We had a limited supply of drugs and only 24 hours in a day and here were thousands of people desperately needing help. At times, I wished there were more hours in a day, as the needs were so great. At other times, when the days had been especially harrowing, with many deaths, I wanted a shorter day, as I was exhausted. On days like that I prayed that tomorrow would be better. But often, it was worse.

When a Somali worker told us many seriously ill children had died during the night, we felt relieved; those kids had left Hell on Earth and were now free from pain and suffering. Because of my Western upbringing, I felt guilty for having such thoughts. My western training said I had to strive to maintain life at all costs and it was clear to see that these innocent children were loved by their parents, who felt just as much grief and pain as any grieving parent losing a child in the West. But somehow, in Somalia, it was different. In those horrendous conditions, it was survival of the fittest. Nature was in control, and she would continue to be so long after the medical teams had gone.

'I look after my healthy child,' a young mum told me one day. 'The sick one will die and so my future is in the healthy one.'

Was this wrong, I wondered? My Western thinking led me to believe this was morally wrong, but the longer I stayed in Somalia, the more I understood the validity of their beliefs and value systems; which were their way of coping in this dreadful situation.

Every morning, we conducted outpatient clinics which I found challenging in the beginning. Hundreds of people would line up, many of whom would not survive to the next day. We became resigned to the fact that we could only do so much with limited staff and drugs. We had no x-ray machine and no laboratory as such, only basic stethoscopes, and for me, the skills for diagnosing that Dr Robin Briant had taught me in Thailand. I had learnt a few Somali words but had to rely heavily on my interpreter, Abdi, whose English was quite basic. The people arrived with symptoms and conditions, and we had to try and figure out what was wrong with them. Many times, I silently cried to God, 'What is wrong with this person?' and a diagnosis would pop into my mind. David Werner's book, *Where There is No Doctor*, became my medical Bible, which I used to help me answer these questions, and I never left the compound without it. Some years later, I had the privilege of meeting David at a course he was running in England, and I was able to thank him for his wonderful and life-saving book.

I'm convinced now that it was only my Christian faith and my awareness of God that kept me going in Somalia. God had called me, and He had promised to equip me. But when dealing with death daily, on such an enormous scale, it's easy to wonder if there are such things in the world as health and life, and hope. At times I wondered how the Somali people ever survived in this remote and barren environment. For them, food was scarce, water was hard to find, and when they did find water it was polluted. There was also the constant threat of the local rebel groups coming into our camp to round up able bodied men and take them off in trucks to fight in the conflicts which were happening in different parts of their country. They did have aid; the World Food programme trucked in food and, working with the Somali Camp officials, rations were handed out to the refugees on a regular basis. These consisted of flour, sugar, oil and sometimes milk powder. Occasionally during my time in the camp, several camels would be slaughtered, and camel meat would be given out to all in the camp, including us if we wanted to try it. The rations may have been meagre, but at least they were there, for the refugees and workers alike.

In those early days at Las Dhure camp, our food was very basic. We had bread, eggs, pasta some tinned meat, and some food we brought out from Hargeisa. I once went on a trip to Djibouti to get supplies with other World Vision staff and we came back to camp with a variety of tinned fruit, tinned vegetables and some fresh fruit and meat from the well-stocked stores we found there. It was like Christmas! Things improved a little over time. Over the months that followed, as our World Vision team grew, the variety of food improved as supplies came in from Nairobi. Even the stores in Hargeisa began to stock food items the Westerners working in the camps there were used to. Despite these basic needs being met, it was incredibly tough in those early days. I felt so isolated, especially when the doctor decided that he had had enough and left, leaving just nurses and a nutritionist in the camp. I began to wonder if there was anyone outside who really cared about us. With pressing needs all around, and the death rate climbing, I wondered at times how long I could keep going before collapsing.

It was the feeling of responsibility that came with our work that could be most challenging. Mothers brought their dying children to us and we alone would have to decide what to do. With limited drugs, limited staff and limited equipment, we had to focus on the children who, with some help, would make it, even if they probably wouldn't reach their second or third birthday. Many, many times we had to tell the mothers that there was nothing more that we could do. In cases like this I would pray in my heart, asking God to take this child to be with Him quickly. Many times, my prayer was answered. At times, words like hope seemed to be in a foreign language, and impossible to hold on to. Somalia certainly wasn't a place for the faint-hearted.

At the end of the day, as the sun was setting and another full day of clinics was over, I would pack up and head back to the compound, to my tent. As I left the clinic, there would still be mothers sitting outside with their seriously ill babies. As I walked past them heading to our compound, completely exhausted, they would grab hold of my trousers, pulling on them and begging me to help them, begging me to look at their critically ill child. I just didn't have anything left inside me; I was totally spent. I was distraught because I knew many of the children would not survive the night, but I also knew that if I didn't leave and get some rest and some sleep I wouldn't be able to return to the clinic and work the following day, and the next day, and the next.

A Bible verse which is found in Matthew, chapter 9: verse 36 says: 'Jesus, when he saw the crowds, he had compassion on them.' I was seeing the crowds, thousands of them, but at times the number of people overwhelmed me. They all were needing some sort of assistance, but there we were so few of us and we couldn't help everyone. It was so hard walking past them all and I felt so torn. As a nurse, I was taught to look after the sickest patient first. But where was I to start, when I was faced with so many sick people? I wanted to show the compassion that Christ had shown, but at times I just couldn't. It was a constant dilemma. Gradually, over the next few weeks, we managed to get some more nurses and doctors, which was a wonderful relief.

19. Midwifery in Somalia: What Challenge Can Teach Us

Being one of the midwives in the camp, I was also involved in obstetrics. We understood that even though the outpatient clinics closed in the late afternoon for the day, we were still on call for the traditional birth attendants should they need us during the night. They only called for help for complex deliveries or when things went wrong. Many nights, the guard would come and call me to go and help a labouring woman somewhere in the camp. I always had to have enough reserves of strength to crawl out of my camp stretcher in the early hours of the morning and go to help a young Somali woman give birth. Out in the camp, miles from any hospital, it was my skills that she and the traditional birth attendants were relying on, at any time of day or night. What pressure that created! With so much death all around, the safe delivery of a healthy baby, especially a boy, brought much celebration to the mother and her family.

Traditional birth attendants (TBAs) – wise women whose skills had been handed down from generation to generation – delivered most of the babies. Their ways were of course very different from what I had learnt during my midwifery course in New Zealand, but I was a guest in their country, and needed to be sensitive to them, their customs, and their cultural practices. During my first few days in Las Dhure, I became aware of the practice of female circumcision, a common custom in this part of the world, but something which was foreign to me. I had never heard about it and it wasn't talked about during either my nursing or midwifery training. Female circumcision is the ritual cutting or removal of some or all the external female genitalia. In Western countries this is often referred to as female genital mutilation. Many countries have tried to ban this, but it is still common practice in several countries around the world today.

The first circumcised woman I saw left me speechless. I found it hard to understand why this practice was considered normal. Later, I was even more surprised when my male interpreter asked me why I was so shocked. 'Aren't all women circumcised?' he asked. 'Certainly not!' I said. 'This doesn't happen where I come from.'

Over the following months, other expatriate midwives and I worked closely with the traditional birth attendants, listening to their experiences and getting to know their traditions. We also shared some of our practices with them. It was a delicate balance of working alongside them, acknowledging their skills and experience and gaining their trust. I was a guest in their country who wouldn't be staying there; they would, and we needed to have a mutual trust and understanding to look after our patients together. Female circumcision was a very sensitive topic amongst our team members in Somalia and although I found the practice not something that I would support, it wasn't my place to criticise their cultural practices. I remember discussing it with one of my African colleagues in Somalia; one day, this person said to me, 'Why do you, as westerners, abort your babies, and put your old people into institutional homes? We don't do that in our culture. Don't criticise the practices you find in some African countries, until you have addressed some of your own practices, which we don't agree with.' Even today, these words ring in my ears.

One of the things I tried to share was hygiene. I stressed to the TBAs the need for handwashing before examining a woman in labour, saying, 'This is very important to reduce infections.' There was no such thing as hand gel back then and water was a scarce commodity. Women spent a good part of their day walking for miles to collect dirty, yellow, contaminated water for cooking and drinking. They often had to dig down into the riverbed for two or three metres with their bare hands to find water and scoop it out into old tin cans. Carefully balancing the tin can on their heads or shoulders, they would make the long journey home. Because wood was so scarce in the area around the camp, they normally didn't boil their drinking water, resulting in the contaminated water being drunk and contributing to the cycle of illness, including diarrhoea and vomiting. The only time when the water was boiled was when they were cooking food.

Purple Hands

The lack of water was brought home to me one night when I was called to help a woman in labour, along with my male interpreter. I could hear high-pitched screaming and wailing coming from her plastic-covered hut. Stooping to enter, I found fifteen women, many of whom were TBAs, making deafening high-pitched sounds as they squatted around the patient. They apparently believed the more noise they made, the quicker the baby would come. The patient was squatting on the dirt floor in great distress. I looked around for water to wash my hands. The women just looked at me as I mimed handwashing. One woman shook her head, signalling there was no water. This was a dilemma; when I conducted training sessions with the TBAs, I was always stressing the need to wash hands before and after delivery. I quickly thought about what I could use and, opening my medical kit, I found a bottle of gentian violet, a bright purple antiseptic dye. I poured some of the liquid into my palm and washed my arms and hands as best I could. In the lantern light, my arms looked like two strange purple appendages. This wasn't in my New Zealand midwifery book!

Through my interpreter, who was outside the hut, I asked the woman to lie down on her back so I could examine her, and I sent up an 'arrow' prayer, 'Please help me, God.' With fifteen pairs of eyes affixed on me, I palpated the woman's swollen abdomen with my purple hands and listened to the foetal heartbeat. I tried to examine her vaginally but as she had extensive scarring from circumcision, it was a challenge. The woman's contractions were getting stronger and the scar tissue was preventing the birth of the baby. I yelled out to my interpreter who relayed the message that I needed to anaesthetise the area, as I was going to have to cut her in order to deliver the baby.

I made a moderate incision with surgical scissors and told the woman to push. After a few massive pushes, the baby's head appeared. The noise in the hut was deafening as the woman's friends screamed and let out high pitched cries at the top of their voices. I carefully untangled the umbilical cord from around the baby's neck and safely delivered a healthy baby boy. The baby began to cry and the noise volume from the women present rose dramatically.

I then proceeded to repair the episiotomy watched by the TBAs who kept trying to help me do the stitching by placing their hands on mine. I sent a stern word out to my interpreter, who told the women that I knew what I was doing so please let me finish the delivery. I then packed up my gear, thanked everyone, received many hugs and smiles from the local TBAs, and my interpreter escorted me back to the camp. That was the first of many complex deliveries I was called to assist with while I was in Las Dhure. What a good night's work!

Back at our tent, I collapsed fully clad on my camp stretcher bed. By torch light I looked down at my purple hands and arms and I smiled to myself. What a steep learning curve that had been, my first delivery of a circumcised woman, having to adapt my normal delivery practice to ensure that both the mother and the baby were safely delivered. I also learned that in a situation where I didn't have gloves, and there was no water, gentian violet was okay. The purple arms and hands gradually faded over the next few days, but were a reminder that this life is all about adapting to whatever comes our way; that we shouldn't be afraid to follow our instincts and training, or to do what we can in this world.

Years later, as I remember that delivery, I still remember my purple hands and arms, and have decided to call my book *Purple Hands*. I have chosen this title to honour the thousands of traditional birth attendants around the world, who continue to deliver millions of babies, in extremely remote villages, clinics and rural hospitals, often under-resourced and frequently without water, persevering with their work despite a serious lack of the essential equipment which we in the West take for granted.

20. Wind, Rain, and Other Acts of Nature

Our living conditions at the camp offered many challenges. We were housed in tents in an extremely harsh climate with very cold temperatures at night and hot, dusty conditions during the day. One terrible night, a fierce storm blew our tent down. My friend and I were up in the middle of the night in our track pants and tops, desperately trying to push tent pegs back into the ground. We got soaked in the pouring rain and spent the night huddled under our damp blankets on our camp stretcher beds, waiting for the morning. Nights like this did not help morale. Living, sleeping and eating in close quarters with people from all corners of the globe was also tough at times, as was the working environment. Under this kind of strain, the very different personalities on our team came to the forefront. We had regular team meetings which helped to sort out some of the concerns, but often the solution was for people to take some time out, and either head to the team house in Hargeisa or fly down to Nairobi for some rest and relaxation.

After a week to ten days on duty in the camp, some of the other team members and I would travel to Hargeisa to have a few days off at one of the two World Vision team houses, while other team members worked at the camp. Sometimes these houses had power and running water, sometimes not, and the plumbing left much to be desired. Once, one of my colleagues flushed the toilet and the entire contents came up through the bath plug hole. We sent the guard to get some help, but he didn't return; instead, this practical girl from New Zealand took steps to fix the problem. Armed with a spade, gloves and a mask, a long piece of wire, disinfectant, a suction cup and much prayer, I set to, desperately recalling basic plumbing principles I'd learnt on my Bible college course. I managed to unblock the toilet and seal the plug hole in the bath. At least it was a change from my usual duties.

When we weren't solving domestic problems, we spent our days off resting, sleeping, writing letters and enjoying a welcome break from our relentless camp duties.

21. Christmas in a Refugee Camp

My first and only Christmas in Somalia was a deeply moving experience. We'd heard that hundreds of refugees were being trucked into the camp on that day. We would need to screen them and hand over blankets, before the commander of the camp arranged for them to have some food rations and plastic sheeting. Early on Christmas morning, we drove up to an area in the camp where the new refugees were arriving. It was a wet morning and bitingly cold. The refugees had nothing but the clothes they stood up in. Many were sick and many of the children were malnourished and extremely unwell. We got started with the screening process. Our medical team members worked alongside the Somali medical helpers, taking aside those who were obviously ill and assessing them as best we could. We gave rations to those who were physically more able and directed them to the camp, where they were shown an area where they could build their shelters.

The triage was a gruelling process, but gradually the rain stopped, and the sun came out. Our next task became my special memory of that day;

handing out blankets and seeing the grateful smiles on the faces of the people who received them. It was as if we'd given them a million dollars, and not just an ordinary grey blanket. For them it meant practical warmth. For me it was an opportunity to show Christian love in that bleak, harrowing situation on Christmas morning. Some women, on receiving their blankets, began making high pitched joyous sounds that pierced the morning air. Some grabbed us and hugged us with tears rolling down their faces, and we found it hard to hold back our own tears.

Later that day, as we made our way back to the team house in Hargeisa for our Christmas dinner, I couldn't help but reflect on the true meaning of Christmas and God's gift of His son Jesus Christ to our world. Although we came from vastly different ethnic and religious backgrounds, we were all human beings and barriers were broken down on that Christmas day. Tears and smiles demonstrated the true meaning of love to every person who was there that day.

Our Christmas dinner consisted of boiled spaghetti, bread, and Fanta. Our Christmas tree was a bare branch decorated with cotton-wool snow. These were all the physical symbols of good tidings we had to celebrate that special day in a place not far away from Bethlehem, just across the Red Sea, where the first Christmas took place more than two thousand years ago. It was probably the most memorable Christmas I've ever had.

The Christmas respite was short-lived. Refugees continued to flood into the various camps, often on the back of trucks, and were usually in a very bad way. Malnutrition was a huge problem, together with common illnesses such as pneumonia, malaria, dysentery, and burns – especially involving children who had fallen into cooking fires. During the months that followed, we slowly set up feeding programmes for severely malnourished children and began to see positive changes.

Teach a Man to Fish…

A major highlight of this assignment for me was assisting an Australian doctor in the trachoma eye operation programme. Trachoma is highly contagious and is the leading preventable cause of blindness in the world. The disease almost always affects both eyes: symptoms begin with mild itching before infection of the eyelashes results in the lashes inverting and rubbing on the eye. If this is not treated, it can lead to blindness. Antibiotics are used to treat early-stage trachoma, but surgery is required in later stages. Access to clean water and improved sanitation are the key to prevention. Because of the prevalence of the condition, we put a great deal of effort into combating it. At the start of the programme, Doctor Ann, a very skilled doctor from Australia, and I were flown down to Mogadishu for two days of training with an eye specialist from England. We then returned to Las Dhure Camp to set up our surgery in a white tent. Our operating table was a door panel placed on empty diesel drums and we had supplies of local anaesthetic and a small stove to boil our surgical instruments. The eye specialist had given us a handy reference manual on how to carry out the operation, and two Somali teenagers who spoke a little English became our interpreters. As we worked with our World Vision Somali health workers and officials, we began to identify countless refugees who needed the basic trachoma eye operation. We soon realised there were too many for the two of us to treat. So, over the following months we trained our two interpreters; prior to our arrival in the camp the young men had been nomads wandering the desert with their parents and a few cows, and now they were becoming capable 'eye doctors!' We supervised them initially as they carried out the operations on their people, and eventually left them to practice on their own. I don't know where they are today; perhaps working in a hospital somewhere in Somalia.

Our public health team also introduced a trachoma prevention programme into the camp. All the children who came to the feeding centres situated around the camp were taught how to wash their eyes and hands before coming inside with a very small amount of the precious water. The combination of flies, dust and dry heat led to many eye infections, and establishing this routine was a relatively simple way of preventing more infection. In our work, we tried as much as we could to pass on preventive practices which could be taught to others by our patients, in the hope they would then pass them on to even more people. In this way, we could extend the range of our care further than the limited resources at our camp would allow.

I learned quite a bit from many of the Somali people we worked alongside in the camp. I found them to be a very proud race of people, who didn't consider themselves to be African, but instead very much Somali. Once, the young Somali men that I worked with told me that all camels in the world belonged to the Somali people; gradually over many years, the camels have spread across the world, but they all originated in Somalia, they informed me. There were many stories such as this one and a sense of shared pride in their ancient origins and culture.

The Somali women, like so many women I met while working on the African continent, had a strong desire to give their children a better life and did their best to do so. They worked alongside us as we set up feeding programmes for the thousands of malnourished children and babies we had in Las Dhure, and worked nonstop in other places throughout the camp, too; collecting wood for the fires so the high protein porridge could be made, walking off early in the morning to dig holes in the often dry river beds to find water, rarely stopping in their efforts to do what was needed for the children in the camp.

The Somali traditional birth attendants I worked with were another vital part of the community, playing the role of the wise older women. They were also handed the mandate to ensure the Somali custom of female circumcision was performed on the young girls. Despite personally really struggling with this ancient cultural practice, I couldn't make any in-roads to change it but learnt to accept that this happened in this part of the world. It wasn't possible, as a guest there, to change it. Male circumcision was also practiced, and I personally saw more young boys coming into the outpatient clinics with infected wounds than I saw young circumcised girls. We did our jobs and tended these patients' needs. Despite obvious differences in our cultures, and our practices, our shared goal of relieving some of the suffering of the inhabitants of that camp was something we were all fully committed to.

22. New Year's Eve in Nairobi, 1980

In the early days in Somalia, when there were only a very few of us, we had some non-medical people who lived in the camp with us and in our team house. These folks from countries all around the world came from a variety of backgrounds and professions, such as engineering and logistics. We would sit outside our tents at night and talk, surrounded by the eighty thousand people who also lived out their lives in the camp; people singing, dancing, crying, yelling at each other, attending the weddings taking place, people dying and babies being born. Sitting out in the middle of the desert under the stars, with only a kerosene lamp, the heartbeat of the camp was audible all around. At times there may have been only two of us workers there under the stars by our tents; at other times there would be more. We would drink tea and share our life stories, our dreams and our struggles. These were precious moments, and often served as an unofficial, necessary debrief, especially if it had been a very tough day, as it often was. This time together helped to keep us sane, caught up as we were in a world of tragedy and pain that was unfolding in front of us every single day.

The aid workers at the camp came from many different places, but we obviously had a great deal in common, be it our calling to be there, or simply our shared experience in that environment. We all became close in the short time we spent together, but there was one special team member I got to know really well during my time in Las Dhure – I will call him Paul (not his real name). We spent many hours listening to each other's stories and sharing from the depths of our hearts. The conversation would often focus on the events taking place all around us; we constantly wondered what was going to happen to all these people. Would peace ever come to this place which the world seemed to have forgotten? These were very heavy conversations for such young people to have, but we were living in an intense time of our lives.

One day, Paul became very ill. We took him back to our house and some other team members and I cared for him. There were several discussions as to whether we should get him out to Nairobi or continue to nurse him where we were. The doctor felt it was better to keep him with us. Gradually, over several weeks he began to recover. During the time I spent nursing him, we had grown closer to each other and as he grew stronger, we talked about the possibility of heading to Nairobi and then out on safari for a few days. It had been an intense situation for me as well, nursing and caring for a special person who was extremely ill, and we both needed a break.

Finally, Paul was well enough to fly, and off we went. Our first few days in Nairobi (where World Vision had got us much appreciated special rates for our accommodation) were quiet. We spent some truly wonderful time together, doing things like relaxing on a veranda watching the sun go down and sipping long, cool drinks before joining others in the dining room for beautiful meals. It was a breathtakingly beautiful place, a complete contrast to the camp in Somalia. When Paul had regained his strength, we booked the safari and the next day we were driven out to the game park.

The Safari camp where we stayed was stunning; a beautiful modern hotel, with lovely grounds, comfortable lounges, delicious food, refreshing swimming pools and areas where people could just sit and relax, sipping cool drinks. Guests sat on comfortable chairs around the swimming pool and wild animals like elephants, different kinds of antelopes, monkeys and the odd water buffalo would wander by. The early rising time for the dawn safari ride ensured that the evening wasn't late, and most of the guests retired to their beds, to be refreshed and ready for the game viewing planned for the next day. We would return from our early morning safari and spend the rest of the day relaxing beside the pool. It was like being on another planet, compared with where we had come from. Our two nights and three days there were just what the doctor ordered.

We happily returned to our pleasant hotel in Nairobi for two more nights, knowing time would go quickly and we'd soon be returning to the dust and grime of Las Dhure, to our tents, the pit latrines and the demands of working in such a stressful environment. On this trip, we were staying in a hotel not far from the Norfolk Hotel, which was a very old and beautifully kept colonial hotel, decorated with photos of famous guests who'd stayed there over the years. The hotel was popular with Kenyans, both white and black, as well as tourists, who could afford the high rates. That night, it was New Year's Eve and a small group of us decided to head out for a meal. We found a restaurant near the Norfolk Hotel, and enjoyed a pleasant evening. Fairly late in the evening we decided to head back to our hotel and watch the fireworks display from our rooms. We were walking along the street, chatting and laughing, wondering what this New Year would bring for us all.

Without warning, there was a huge explosion, with clouds of dust shooting into the air and a strong smell of something burning. We were thrown to the ground, with glass from the shop windows shattering all around us. Our first thoughts were that something must have happened at the Norfolk Hotel. Amidst the noise, the smoke and the confusion, it was hard to work out where the explosion had come from. Luckily, none of us was hurt. We scrambled to our feet, and keeping close together, hurried back to our hotel, which fortunately had been left unscathed. We were mightily relieved to be away from the flames, the shouting and the agonised cries of the wounded. Sitting in a room high up in the multi-storey hotel, we watched the confusion as ambulance and police sirens blasted the dusty night air. We switched on the TV. The local announcer was pleading with viewers to go and donate blood, to help the many people who'd been badly injured. At that stage nobody knew exactly how many people had been killed. We were grateful that we'd all escaped injury, as this was later confirmed as a terrorist attack. As midnight came, and the old year rolled over for the new year to take its place, we began to wonder what 1981 had in store for us all. We felt grateful to God that we were safe while we prayed for those who were seriously injured and for the families of those who had been killed.

This was the report in the Kenyan *Daily Nation* newspaper the next day.

> That night, New Year's Eve in 1980, a bomb flattened the Norfolk Hotel in Nairobi, killing 20 people and injuring 80. Responsibility for the attack was claimed by an Arab group that said it was seeking retaliation for Kenya's allowing Israeli troops to refuel in Nairobi during the raid on Entebbe Airport in Uganda four years earlier to rescue hostages from a hijacked aircraft.
>
> According to reports about that incident, international security agencies in conjunction with the Kenyan Police had a prime suspect within hours. He was identified as 34-year-old Qaddura Mohammed Abdel al-Hamid of Morocco, and he was said to have checked into the Norfolk Hotel in Nairobi in the last week of 1980. Al-Hamid was found to have paid for his room up until New Year's Day but slipped away on the afternoon of 31 December. He had boarded a plane for Saudi Arabia by the time the guests at the Norfolk assembled for a New Year's Eve dinner.

23. More Adventures Await

After our refreshing, if upsetting, time in Kenya, we returned to Somalia and back to our work in the refugee camp. One day, Paul came to me with some disturbing news. He was being sent to another camp in the south of Somalia, a very long way from Las Dhure camp, as his skills were needed there. It was tough saying our good-byes. We knew we'd have to resort to letter writing as our main form of communication, there being no such things as cell phones then. Nor was there a postage service in Somalia – we had to rely on someone taking our letters and posting them overseas. In our case, though, it was a matter of ensuring that the United Nations plane that flew to South Somalia would take the mail, and hopefully bring it to the World Vision Office in the capital city, where it would be put on the Somali Airlines flights to Hargeisa

Over the months that followed, Paul suggested that I come and visit him. Fortunately, I had some leave owing and was keen to make the trip. I managed to get a flight to Mogadishu and then a seat on the UN plane to the south, which carried aid workers, supplies and mail. Since Somalia is such a big country, the plane would stop at many little airfields along the way, dropping people off and collecting people and supplies. I boarded the plane, having been given the name of the stop where I needed to disembark. We passengers introduced ourselves to each other and chatted companionably as we took off. We seemed to have been travelling for hours, having already made several stops, when I finally got off, along with a couple of other passengers. The pilot unloaded the luggage and waved good-bye. The people who were dropped off with me asked me if someone was meeting me. 'Yes,' I said, 'my friend Paul giving them his full name. They knew him, but the look on their faces disturbed me deeply. 'What's wrong?' I asked, with a tight feeling in my stomach. I'd been certain this was the right stop. 'Barbara,' they said, 'you've got off the plane three stops too early and there's no other way to get there. The plane doesn't travel to where Paul is until next week. I was terribly upset at having made such an idiotic mistake. I stood there, in shock, desperately trying to work out what I could do. 'Come back to our base; we'll look after you until we can work something out,' they suggested, and I had no option but to accept their kind offer. I felt such a fool. How could I have been so stupid? I was a couple of hours from where he was and there was no way I could get to him.

Later that afternoon, I was able to talk to Paul over the radio. After his initial dismay at hearing what happened, we laughed about it, despite our frustration that it wasn't going to be possible to meet up. I spent three days with my new friends before catching the plane back to Mogadishu airport. The morning I was due to fly out, I picked up a stomach bug, which made my flight back to the capital exceptionally uncomfortable. There was no toilet on the UN plane. It was a matter of hanging on and hoping I'd make it. Around two hours later, we landed at the airport. I was desperate by then, getting more and more agitated as our plane seemed to take forever to taxi to an area a long way from the basic terminal building. When the door finally opened to let us off, I raced down the stairs of the plane. With not a toilet in sight, I found a private area behind a shed. In a situation like that, when you must go you have to go!

Some miserable stories can have a happy ending. I had fourteen hours to spend in the capital, Mogadishu, before flying back to Hargeisa early in the morning, so I stayed the night in Paul's friend's co-worker's house. I hit the bed feeling tired, emotionally as well as physically. I was also feeling very annoyed with myself. In the early hours of the morning, there was a knock on the door and my host got up to see who it was. I couldn't believe my eyes! It was Paul. He'd decided to come so that we could have some time together, even if just a few hours. He told me his story about getting to Mogadishu, which included hitch-hiking, crossing rivers, avoiding the crocodiles, riding in the cab of Somali trucks and finally getting there. It was incredible – and heart-warming! We sat and talked for the rest of the night, before he took me to the airport, and I left him to fly back to the camp.

24. At the Mercy of the Banks of Africa

The next time we were able, Paul and I decided to take a break. We organised a visit to the Seychelles – islands off the coast of Somalia and a favourite destination for aid workers in Somalia – although this wasn't straightforward; few things were, in that part of the world in those days. We'd arranged our flights and accommodation through a travel agent in Nairobi and went to the main bank in Mogadishu to buy foreign currency, ideally American dollars. The man behind the counter told us to wait, and soon we were ushered into the bank manager's office. He had reasonable English, so we explained to him what we were wanting. 'No problems,' he said with a smile. 'We are short of foreign currency at the moment as the President has taken one of our two Somali Airlines planes and most of our foreign currency and gone to a meeting of African leaders. What I can do is write you a letter. When you get to the Seychelles, go into this bank and the bank manager will be able to help you.'

Looking back how, naïve we were!

A few days later, we arrived in the Seychelles and checked into our rooms. We then decided to head to the bank and change some of our Somali money. When arrived at the bank we asked to see the bank manager, as we'd been directed by the Somali bank manager, who invited us to sit, and asked how he could help us. We explained our situation and handed him the letter from the bank manager in Somalia. He read it and tore it up, saying, 'I'm sorry but this letter is worthless. We are getting so many of them. I'm sorry, but I can't help you.' He asked who we were working for, and when we told him, he thought for a moment and said, 'I can do this for you. If you contact your offices in Nairobi and ask them to send a bank draft to us, I can arrange for you to get some Seychelles currency.' We had no choice. I gave him my details and he handed me his phone. I called the World Vision office in Nairobi, who arranged for money to be transferred to the bank in the Seychelles. The Bank Manager told us to come back later in the day, and, true to his word, he had the money waiting for us. How delighted we were, despite the incredible hassles we had to go through to do the simplest things. Being adaptable is possibly the foreign aid workers' strongest skill!

We spent ten lovely days in the Seychelles, relaxing and recovering from our time in Somalia (apart from being robbed, and Paul's camera being stolen, incidents we had no choice but to brush off, and learn from). On our return to Somalia, we went back to see that bank manager, who uncompromisingly said to us, 'If the bank manager in the Seychelles won't accept my letter and my request, then it is his problem, not mine,' while ushering us out of his office. Paul returned to his camp and I to mine, both having learned a bit more about the way's things work in Somalia!

Over the next few weeks, for a variety of reasons, Paul and I decided to stop writing. It was a mutual arrangement; I carried on in my work and he persevered with his. Years later, he married and returned to Africa to continue his missionary work. Our paths never crossed again.

25. Up in the Air, and in God's Hands

During the year I spent in Somalia, traveling for work or heading to Nairobi on holidays always involved having to fly, usually on the regular Somali Air flights between Hargeisa and Mogadishu. We were not allowed to travel by land from Hargeisa because of the on-going conflict between Ethiopia and Somalia. The thing was, I didn't like flying! This fear stemmed from several near misses I had experienced while flying around Africa, in planes ranging from jets to two-seater aircraft. I had two close shaves in Somalia and to this day I still pray fervently when I fly. All the aid workers shared these concerns, but we just had to fly anyhow, and place ourselves in God's hands.

Our worst fears were confirmed one day when we heard the news that a Somali Airline plane had crashed en route from Mogadishu to Hargeisa. A new nurse from Uganda who had been coming to join our medical team was on that plane. We'd been busy preparing for her arrival but sadly, she never arrived; everyone on board was killed. Our hearts went out to her family and friends in Uganda. (We found out later that there were several high-ranking Somalian military generals on board the plane on that day, along with some other civilian passengers, and investigations concluded that a bomb had been planted on the plane.) The death of our new worker also hit us all very hard as we had all flown that route ourselves and knew the dangers every time we flew.

I'll never forget one of these particularly hair-raising flights, when two expatriate doctors and I were returning from a meeting in Mogadishu. The plane was coming into land at Berbera Airport, about two and a half hours by road from Hargeisa. During our descent, we were going at such a speed that I could see the end of the runway fast approaching through my cabin window. As the ground rapidly loomed, I could feel the Somalian passengers around me becoming agitated, sensing something was seriously wrong. Aghast, my colleagues and I grabbed each other's hands, thinking our time was up. Suddenly, the pilot decided to abort the landing. He threw the plane straight upwards with such force that we were pinned back against our seats. No-one spoke as the pilot completed a circuit, descended, and made a successful landing. We stayed in our seats for some time, struggling to regain our composure. When we disembarked, we collapsed on the tarmac, shaking uncontrollably. Our team leader, who was waiting on the tarmac, helped us up. Having witnessed the aborted landing, he hugged us sympathetically, before driving us back to the camp at Hargeisa. That was a very quiet trip, as the reality of what might have happened sunk in. This close shave did nothing to engender in me any love of flying in Africa.

Another flight I remember vividly took place in 1982, not in Somalia, but in Sudan. World Vision International had asked me to join a small group flying from Nairobi across Sudan to the Chad border, in order to gauge the number of refugees from Chad crossing the border to Sudan.

This was a seven-day fact-finding mission planned in response to the Sudanese government's claim that hundreds of refugees were arriving each day; therefore, they were requesting aid from the international community to assist with the situation.

Our six-member party comprised a female doctor, three men (a wealthy Texan businessman interested in relief work; Joshua, the World Vision International Relief Director; and a World Vision field worker who spoke Sudanese), the pilot, and me. Departing from Nairobi Airport, we began the 3,000 km flight to the city of El Genenia in Western Sudan, across the vast country that was Sudan. During our four-hour flight, we alternately read, slept, and chatted above the drone of the engines. Joshua shared with us stories of the many times his plane had got lost while flying over parts of Africa, causing me more anxiety.

We finally landed in El Genenia and the plane taxied towards a small building. Suddenly, the plane was surrounded by armed tanks and stern-faced soldiers pointing machine guns at us. I was relieved that our World Vision African interpreter could speak Sudanese, and that we had all the required paperwork. The pilot and Joshua quickly presented our passports, visas and landing papers and after much animated discussion, we could disembark. We were told to climb into the Land Cruiser which was on the tarmac and were driven to the Sultan's office.

The office was a very large one-storey white building with a few trees and flowers around the driveway. We got out of the vehicle, and accompanied by an official, were led down long corridors into the Sultan's office. He was a huge man of over seven feet tall and wore a long, white, flowing robe, and a small cap on the back of his head. The Sultan had a good command of English and spoke warmly to us, inviting us to sit on very large and comfortable chairs. We were soon served glasses of strong and extremely sweet tea, so thick that the spoons stood upright in the glass (When the Sultan briefly left his office, we poured the sickly brew into nearby pot-plants. Seeing our empty glasses, he offered to refill them, but we declined his kind offer.) By the time we had settled into this visit, it was early afternoon, and the Sultan finally said he'd arranged for a driver to take us to an area near the Chad border where refugees were known to be crossing. It was a long drive, but we would be stopping en-route for dinner, he assured us. Climbing on board the well-used Land Cruiser, we were driven north.

Purple Hands

On and on we drove, across the desert landscape and into the back of beyond. Lulled by the sound of the engine, we spent most of our time dozing, jolting awake when we hit particularly rough ground. Night fell, and we continued our journey not quite sure where we were going to end up. Suddenly, the driver stopped. It must have been past midnight. We looked around, puzzled. We were in the middle of nowhere. The driver said: 'We'll have some food here.' Wearily we clambered out, wondering where the food would be coming from, not realising the amazing experience we were about to have; figures emerged from the night, bearing baskets of food on their heads. They placed a great variety of meat, bread, and local treats on beautiful carpets and invited us to partake of the feast. We were also offered our favourite sweet tea, before the figures were absorbed back into the darkness. As we sat under the awe-inspiring African sky, I thought, 'This is unreal!' We never did find out who those people were who had shown us such incredible hospitality, but I suspect the Sultan of the area was involved.

The driver signalled it was time to move on and we climbed on board again and took off. It was still pitch dark when we arrived in a small village. The men in our party were dropped at a local 'hotel' and the doctor and I were taken to the local schoolteacher's house to sleep. She invited us inside and signalled that I was to sleep in her bed. I shook my head politely, but she insisted. She woke a woman in another room and offered my colleague her bed. Our hostesses slept on mattresses on the floor. As we climbed into the already-warm beds and drifted off to sleep, I thought, 'This is true hospitality,' and wondered if I would offer my bed to a stranger who arrived at my house at 3.00 am.

We were up again a few hours later, grateful for our brief sleep. We thanked our hostesses and headed further north along the Chad border to where the Chadian refugees were said to be crossing. We arrived in the area and managed to find a tea house and meet with the local leader who took us to the area in question. We spent the day interviewing people in various villages, but to our great surprise we found no refugees. After spending the night in a small guest house, we decided to return to El Genenia in the morning as we hadn't located a single refugee. It was late afternoon when we arrived at the Sultan's office and told him we had found no refugees. The Sultan seemed somewhat surprised and said we must prepare a report for the Sudanese Government. We thanked him for his wonderful hospitality and then drove out to the airport to catch our plane to Khartoum, thinking what an adventure we had all just had, and what stories we had to tell, but little did we know, our adventures had only just begun!

As we flew to Khartoum, the capital of Sudan, unwinding from our experience, our Kiwi pilot suddenly became very ill with vomiting and was so nauseous he couldn't fly the plane. This was nerve-wracking, to say the least. Fortunately, our Texan friend was sitting in the co-pilot's seat and took over the controls. What happened next was truly a miracle. There are no words that can describe our collective joy when our Texan colleague revealed that he owned the same plane back in Texas. Our new pilot managed to radio Khartoum airport and explain our predicament; the airport was immediately closed to all other incoming and outgoing traffic. He circled the runway and began the descent, eventually landing us safely. Very relieved, we gave him quite a round of applause. I can assure you I was glad to put my feet on solid ground, Thank you, God, for Texan pilots.

As was agreed, we met with Sudanese officials who were overseeing the refugee situation and they weren't exactly happy about the fact that we'd not found any refugees. Perhaps they'd been hoping to receive some of the aid funds being poured into African countries for such evacuees. After our meeting, we spent a few days in Khartoum to recover, before our somewhat healthier pilot flew us all safely back to Nairobi.

26. Farewell Somalia, Hello Calcutta

It had been a difficult year for me in Somalia. Working in such a hard, isolated environment and living in a tent in the middle of a desert at the mercy of the heat, sandstorms and rain was tough. Even more, trying to help the thousands of emaciated and dehydrated famine victims with insufficient food, medical supplies and equipment was overwhelming.

Our team was made up of dedicated and talented aid workers from around the world, all committed to making a difference, but each of us struggled at times to believe that we could. Despite the hopelessness I felt at times, by the end of my year in Las Dhure, I did see the wheels of despair and heartache turn towards change and something more positive. Many of the children began to respond to the food that they were receiving regularly during the day, and over time, we saw children who had been displaying all the signs and symptoms of tuberculosis begin to respond to the treatment we gave. Trust between us and the local Somalia staff also strengthened, and the incidence of trachoma began to decrease due to our prevention programmes established in the feeding centres. Further, the surgery we performed on many patients succeeded in removing their pain.

However, sickness continued to strike our own team, making us chronically short of staff and I wasn't immune; it was common for all of us to succumb to diarrhoea and vomiting. Our diet in Somalia was limited to; pasta, very few fresh vegetables, lots of local bread, eggs and occasionally some camel meat which the Somalia Camp Commandant would donate to us. Such conditions affected morale, but more importantly, it affected our physical health, and no one could last too long in the camps. After a while, I knew I was exhausted, had nothing more to give, and was ready to head home, leaving behind part of my heart with the brave people there, but also knowing that I had given my best and it had been worthwhile.

My contract ended around that time and it was time for me to return to New Zealand for a well-earned break before deciding what was next. Ann, an Australian doctor I'd met at the camp, was leaving at the same time, and so we decided to travel together and planned some stops along the way.

Sisters of Mercy

We decided we would travel to Calcutta and work for Mother Teresa's order for ten days, as many people were doing at that time. After flying into Calcutta, we hired a taxi from the airport to our accommodation; a girls' hostel attached to a local school near the Sisters of Mercy, the order founded by Mother Teresa. Fortunately, the hostel had a spare room with two single beds, two chairs and a few clothes hooks on the back of the door with a bathroom down the corridor. We unpacked our things, got some sleep, and the next day we walked down a busy side street to the main house of the Sisters of Mercy.

An Indian nun wearing the order's white headdress and white cotton sari bordered with blue greeted us at the door and welcomed us in. Ann and I explained that we, a doctor and nurse midwife, were on our way home from doing relief work in Somalia and wanted to spend a short time helping Mother Teresa and the nuns in any way we could. She accepted our offer and that afternoon, the nuns took us to the Home of the Destitute and Dying. I don't remember much about what the building looked like on the outside, but as we entered, we saw rows of beds with severely ill people just lying on mattresses in the stifling heat. The home was vastly different from the hospices in Western countries where dying people have modern amenities and private rooms. We were introduced to the Indian nuns who were working in the home and showed us how we could help them and their many patients. We were given a short history about each patient and what medication they were on, and they asked Ann for advice about any patient with a more serious condition. Many of these destitute people had been found lying on the streets, close to death, nameless, and without anyone to care for them. It was an exceedingly grim place to work in, but also a special place because of the love the nuns and volunteers lavished on their patients. Many of the patients received more love and dignity while they lay dying than they had ever received during their lives.

Working alongside the nuns and some of the other volunteers, I washed patients, made beds, helped patients sip water and fanned others, making them as comfortable as possible. The nurses often asked me to sit with a dying person and hold their hand as their life came to an end. What a privilege to comfort a fellow human being at that time. I didn't know the patients' names or language, but I was able to minister to them as one human being to another.

After a few days in the Home for the Dying, we were assigned to a free clinic run by the Sisters of Mercy at the Calcutta railway station. To reach the clinic, we had to make our way through this enormous railway station, already jam-packed with early morning crowds swarming in all directions. Fortunately, we had one of Mother Teresa's Sisters, Agnes, to guide us through the teeming throng.

Keeping Agnes in our sights, we narrowly avoided tripping over bundles of clothing and blankets that were strewn everywhere; we were appalled to learn that masses of people routinely slept in the station overnight. When authorities came to move them on, many were already dead. This was the reality of living in the densely populated city of Calcutta.

Over the next few days, we saw hundreds of patients with a variety of conditions: chest infections, high fevers, skin infections, stomach upsets and eye infections. People came to these clinics because they couldn't afford to go to the doctors' clinics which were all around the railway station. I worked as an assistant for Dr Ann who diagnosed and treated patients as best she could. There were no scans, x-rays or even blood tests, and so Dr Ann made her diagnosis by stethoscope, physical examination and experience. The clinic provided only basic care but served a need which wasn't otherwise being met.

One afternoon, we finished the clinic early and returned to Mother Teresa's main house to attend a simple service of prayer and reflection. Mother Teresa and several of her nuns were already seated on the floor when we quietly sat down to join them. It was a privilege to kneel in the same chapel as this humble Albanian nun whose devotion to serving others led her to become one of the world's most influential people; the tiny woman who had devoted her life to serving the poor and founding the Sisters of Mercy. After a time of both silent and spoken prayer, Mother Teresa stood up, smiled at us, and left the chapel. I pinched myself, realising I'd just joined in prayer with this amazing woman and her dedicated team, all of us asking for God's help and wisdom to continue this ministry of serving the poor and dying in the slums of Calcutta and other parts of India.

One afternoon, we visited a small hospital run by an American doctor. It was set up by the doctor to care for abandoned babies found by the Sisters of Mercy nuns outside abortion clinics in the streets of Calcutta. Many of these babies had been aborted late in pregnancy and, barely alive, were brought to the clinic to be given a chance of life. Most of these premature babies were lying in incubators, row upon row, being cared for by the doctor and his team of nurses. We were told that some of these babies would be adopted, but many others would not find homes and families to belong to and would face an uncertain future. Sadly, walking away from the clinic that day, I thought of the many couples in New Zealand, where very few babies are put up for adoption, longing to adopt a baby. I also reflected on the patients I'd seen in the home for the destitute and dying a few streets away and wondered how many of those babies would struggle to survive and end up spending their last days in that home. Poverty and homelessness form a vicious circle.

During my time overseas, I often thanked God that I was born in New Zealand, as our lives are so blessed compared to the lives of thousands of people I met in countries like India and Africa. Having been given so much, I felt strongly that I must use my training and skills to make a difference. God had equipped me, and I wasn't going to give up, despite any difficult working conditions.

27. Nepal

After our seven-day stint in India, Ann and I flew to Nepal for a brief stay with Kathy Crombie, a former flatmate from my Auckland nursing days. We spent our first night in a mission guest house in Kathmandu, before Kathy met us the next morning to guide us to the mission station where she worked, some distance from Kathmandu. The three of us rose early and headed to the Kathmandu bus station to buy our tickets, thankful that Kathy spoke fluent Nepali. We took the local bus via Pokhara, and after a few hours, clambered off and readied ourselves for the long climb up the track to the mission hospital in Ampipal, situated in the nearby mountain (Fortunately, Kathy had hired Sherpa porters to carry our suitcases as the path was steep and tiring.) We trudged through small villages beautifully cultivated with terraced patterns as the path curved around the side of hills. After several hours of steeper and steeper gradients, we reached our destination in the late afternoon: a small mission hospital with commanding views, built high in the mountains.

We were exhausted but glad to have arrived, despite sore legs and aching feet. Only a few weeks earlier, I'd been in the desert of Somalia, and then the slums of Calcutta; Ampipal was like being in a paradise of snow-capped mountains, green grass, blue skies and clean running streams. This was to be our home for a few days, and it was good to be here, and realise that for a short time we could just be and enjoy this small but beautiful piece of God's creation.

We soon met the staff of the hospital, and after a light tea, climbed into bed and slept soundly, worn out as we were from our day's travelling and so much physical effort. The next day, we were taken on a tour of the hospital, meeting the staff and patients, many of whom had walked for days to come in for treatment. Although it was small and rural, it was very well equipped, with a good selection of medication, trained local doctors and nurses, ex-pat doctors, and an extensive outreach health programme for the surrounding villages. We were there as guests of Kathy, so where she went, we went, observing and learning from her and the other staff. As we wandered around and took it all in, I couldn't help but compare it to the camp in Somalia and the clinics in the slums of Calcutta. The differences were extreme, and I struggled with this, trying to understand the unfairness of this world in which we live.

After our little hiatus at the top of the world, Ann and I spent a few days in Thailand where she visited a friend who was working in one of the refugee camps and I was able to return to the two camps I had previously worked in. Talking with several staff who were working in the camps, it was heart-warming to hear that many of the refugees I had worked with were now on their way to new countries and new lives. This news was so wonderful to me, and I was delighted that I, along with so many other aid workers, had played a part in their second chances. It means so much to us to have happy feedback when our day-to-day work in those places didn't have immutable results. (I was especially fortunate some years later while working in Dunedin to meet a Cambodian woman at the church I was attending. She had some English and I was able to establish that she had spent some time in Khao I Dang while I was there. We hadn't met in the camp, but she was so delighted to find someone who knew where she had been and knew some of the hardships and heart breaks she had seen and been through. The warmth of her hug said it all, but in broken English she added, 'Thank you. You know Khao I Dang.' I smiled and hugged her back, understanding.)

After our brief visits to the camps, Ann and I parted company. She flew home to Australia, and I back to New Zealand, wondering, not for the first time or the last, what God had in store for me next. What I did know was that I needed rest and relaxation in order to recharge myself, both physically and emotionally. Not only was I tired, but I needed time to reflect on and process what I had been through; I had seen so much suffering and pain and I couldn't forget what I had experienced. I had witnessed almost more death than I had life; I had seen the best and worst in human beings; I couldn't imagine anyone taking in any more than what I had in the past few years. Little did I know that in the years to follow, I would see so much more.

28. New Directions:
The World Vision Disaster Response Team

I didn't have long to wait before the next stage began to unfold. World Vision were looking at pulling together a team of expert doctors and nurses who would be on stand-by, ready to respond to disasters around the world at short notice. I fit the bill and was chosen to be a potential member of this proposed team. World Vision paid for me to go to England for a period of training.

I was based in London to start with. My first lot of training was in disaster management and I settled into the course well. I enjoyed the study, finding meeting other aid workers from around the world stimulating. The course looked at all aspects of working in a disaster situation. Topics including food supplies, water and sanitation, medical issues, security, recruiting of staff, communications and inter-agency relationships were all covered. It would have been great to have done this course before I had gone to Thailand, but I was pleased to be doing the course; better late than never.

While in London, I stayed with Chris, a friend I'd worked with in Somalia. He ran a weekly home group and it was lovely to meet with other Christians, to discuss the Bible and relevant issues of the day. I told the group that I'd soon be heading to Liverpool to attend a three-month course at the School of Tropical Medicine and asked if they knew anyone there that I could link up with, as I didn't know a single person in that city. One group member passed on the name of some very good friends of hers. The husband, Roger Derbridge, was vicar of an Anglican Church in Liverpool, and he and his wife Sheila had five children. 'Look them up,' she said, 'They'll look after you.'

Liverpool

The Liverpool School of Tropical Medicine, a registered charity, specialised in promoting improved health and health systems for poor and disadvantaged peoples, especially in developing countries. It was a fascinating place to be. We learnt so much about the diseases I'd already encountered in Somalia, Thailand and Singapore and we studied many other diseases which I had yet to come across. We spent time having lectures, sharing ideas and stories in small groups, and doing practical laboratory work. This lab work involved peering into microscopes, examining urine and faeces from hospital patients who had been admitted following their time overseas. We were looking for worms and other creepy-crawlies. If any of us complained of stomach aches, then what better place than the lab to carry out an examination on one's own body waste!

There were some interesting students in our class, including two of Colonel Gaddafi's nephews, who worked in the Tripoli hospitals as nurses. They rarely attended lectures and seemed to spend a lot of their time trying to recruit us to come and work for them in their hospital. They offered attractive packages which included a house, a car, and of course, a husband.

As part of the course, each of us had to do a presentation to our fellow students. This was supposed to last for twenty minutes and show something of the type of medical work the student had been doing prior to coming to Liverpool. We all dutifully did what we were asked to do, except for the two Libyan boys, who had brought with them the latest propaganda film which was three-quarters of an hour long. The Colonel himself was the main star, and the topic was all about how he was saving the country. The film, as I remember it, was full of promises, guns, tanks, and propaganda that could only have come from Colonel Muammar al-Gaddafi There were many shots of thousands upon thousands of people cheering and seemingly worshipping Gaddafi as he was driven with his huge entourage through the streets of Tripoli. As I watched it, I thought, 'I don't think that is where God is calling me to go...' Gaddafi's two nephews tried very hard to sell us all a deal, but no matter how attractive the package may have been, it certainly wasn't something I was interested in getting into. Such a deal would certainly come with many strings attached, strings that I would have had no control over. Along with every other girl in the class, I politely declined their offers. It is interesting to look back at those days now, in the light of subsequent international political events in Libya!

Going to church can be dangerous

One Sunday while in Liverpool, I decided to go and find St Mary's Anglican Church. I was feeling encouraged to meet these people I'd been told to contact, during my time in London. So, I caught a bus to St Mary's and walked in. My life was about to change. God knew this. He was about to speak to me again.

I was greeted warmly at the door and went and found a seat, smiling at the woman sitting beside me. I was sitting a few rows from the front and sat quietly for a few moments, waiting for the service to begin. Suddenly, a woman came over to me. 'Welcome,' she said, 'My name is Sheila and my husband Roger is the vicar. What is your name and where do you come from?' I said who I was, where I was from, and why I was at church that morning. Her next question was, 'What are you doing for lunch? Please come and join us at the vicarage. We have five children, so it may be a bit noisy, but we would love you to come. I'll catch up with you after the service.' What a wonderful welcome!

The service began with worship very much like I was used to, and I relaxed and enjoyed it very much. During the service, the Vicar asked us all to turn to the person beside us and spend a few minutes asking them about themselves, and then share the peace of God with them. I turned to the woman beside me, asked her name and invited her to tell me a little about herself. Her name was Jo and she was recovering from typhoid, which she'd caught in Pakistan. She was a midwife and had worked on the Afghan-Pakistan border in a place called Bannu. She couldn't return to Bannu and was struggling with that reality, as she had loved the work out there. She told me the hospital in Bannu desperately needed a replacement midwife before turning to me and saying, 'What's your name? What do you do?'

I told Jo my name, explained that I was a nurse-midwife, studying at the School of Tropical Medicine, and that prior to that I'd been working as a nurse midwife in Somalia, in Thailand and on the World Vision boat *Seasweep*. I explained that I hoped to join the World Vision Disaster Team, depending on the next disaster coming along, but if that didn't happen, I didn't have a job. She immediately said, 'Why don't you go to Bannu, in Pakistan? They desperately need a midwife.' It was then that the Vicar called the congregation to order. I don't remember much of the rest of the service, as I was thinking about Bannu in Pakistan, already having conversations in my mind; God smiling, and me being apprehensive. After the service Jo said to me, 'Think about it!' I immediately replied that I didn't have the airfare and wasn't sure how I could get there. 'Don't worry,' she said, taking a piece of paper out of her bag, 'When your course is finished and you head back to London, give these people a ring. They could get you out to Pakistan.' The list had three names, all well-known English mission societies. I thanked her and she left, saying to me, 'God will guide you and take you there if that's what He has in mind for you.'

My head was still spinning when Sheila Derbridge came over and invited me to lunch, saying she would love for me to meet their children. So, off I went with Roger, Sheila and their five kids for a delicious lunch and cheerful family time of getting to know each other. Sheila and Roger and their family became treasured friends. They welcomed me into their family way back then, and they remain close friends today.

The encounter in St Mary's Church was certainly of God, an encounter that was to change the course of my life once again. I completed the course in Liverpool, headed back to London and found that World Vision had no disasters for me to be involved with, so I rang the first name on the mission society list, the Church Missionary Society United Kingdom (CMS UK). I explained who I was, what I'd been doing, and that although World Vision couldn't use me right now, I was desperate for a job. I'm not sure what I was expecting, but the reaction I got was surprising!

'This is amazing!' declared the voice on the end of the phone. 'You are an answer to prayer. We've just received an urgent request from the obstetrician in Bannu. The hospital is desperately short of midwives. We have literally just finished praying. When can you come in and see us?' 'I can catch a tube train in an hour, and see you at 1:00 pm,' I replied in nonchalant Kiwi style. The man seemed a bit surprised; I later found out the British usually make appointments for a few days' time.

Arriving at the mission headquarters that afternoon, I was introduced to several people on the board and they invited me to a forthcoming selection weekend in the East End of London. I accepted and soon went through a thorough vetting process, along with other applicants, that would help to decide who was suitable for the posting and who was not. During the weekend, each candidate was observed, questioned and interviewed by a psychologist, a counsellor, and a doctor. I was asked many questions about my upbringing, my nursing and midwifery training, my theological training and my commitment to Christ. We all observed periods of silence, and I spent much time praying about this new adventure: I only wanted to go where God wanted me to be. I learned that Bannu was an isolated place and that my life there would be far from easy. On the Sunday afternoon, I had my final session with the selection panel. They were happy to accept me to go to Bannu Hospital but felt that I needed more preparation. They felt my missionary training in Australia had been a bit narrow, and that I needed to gain a wider view of different aspects of what I would call more liberal theology, before heading to Pakistan, recommending I spend six weeks at the CMS training school in Birmingham.

Still undecided, I returned to where I was staying in London, where I spent the next few days praying and reflecting on my future. Eventually, my mind made up, I rang CMS and accepted their conditions. I would go to Bannu, Pakistan as a midwife, initially for two years and then review my options. The society planned for me to travel to Birmingham, to join another Kiwi I had met many years ago in Auckland, a man called Warren Parker, who was heading out to Tanzania. We spent the next six weeks attending lectures, walking across snow-covered grass to the heated swimming pool nearby and generally having a wonderful, relaxing time. With our accommodation and food paid for, we were given a small allowance of one pound a day, which limited our socialising, but was enough to get us by. The six weeks passed quickly, while I attended lectures of my choice each day, worked and studied with other students, went to workshops on the cross cultural aspects of mission work, and on Sundays, joined services at the very different African and West Indian churches dotted around Birmingham, a highlight for me.

Returning to London, I soon was busy with medical checks, vaccinations and last-minute packing. I found the farewell service rather unsettling, though. As a Kiwi going out with CMS UK, I wasn't regarded as British and so wasn't included when the CMS British people were commissioned. What's more, despite being a Kiwi, I wasn't commissioned with my friend Warren either. I was in no man's land and felt very left out. However, my continuing comfort was that God had called me to go to Bannu, and for me His commissioning was fine for me. Prior to heading overseas to Pakistan, I was allocated three churches in the United Kingdom which would become my link churches. The parishioners would pray for and support me, and I would write to them while I was away to keep them up-to-date with my work. Whenever I was back in England, I would visit them, too. In being a part of this exchange, I met truly wonderful people, some of whom I am still in contact with today.

The rest, as they say, is history. I was about to be on my way to Pakistan, as the first New Zealander ever to live in Bannu, a cantonment town in the north-west frontier province of Pakistan, bordering Afghanistan. Prior to the partition of India and Pakistan in 1947, Bannu had been a British Military Post, with the Pennell Memorial Hospital located outside the city walls in the 'army cantonment area,' a name that continued after the partition.

Yet another adventure awaited!

29. New Culture, New Location, New Challenges

Pennell Memorial Hospital, North-West Frontier Province, Pakistan

It was early morning when I was warmly met at Islamabad Airport by Beryl, a middle-aged British woman, who greeted me with a big smile and bigger 'Welcome!' I noticed immediately that she was wearing baggy trousers and a long shirt; her version of the shalwar kameez, national dress of Pakistan. I knew this because I had, thankfully, supplied myself in London with some real shalwar and kameez, as well as a dupatta, the scarf worn across the front of the kameez. I really enjoyed wearing these items of clothing and took them with me to all the places I worked following my time in Pakistan because they were so comfortable, and practical in the many situations I found myself in where modesty was needed. Even more helpfully, I realised as I looked around me at the thousands of others at the airport dressed similarly, I fitted right in! As we walked through the airport, about to embark on my latest adventure, Beryl assured me that, 'the Bannu ladies are looking forward to having you join them!' I wondered who on earth the Bannu ladies were as we negotiated the crowds and hoped that I would fit in with them, too.

After collecting my bags, Beryl briskly led the way to a nearby Land Rover and the patiently waiting Pakistani chauffeur. With my luggage safely stored, and wondering what was in store for me next, I climbed into the back seat, searching in vain for a seatbelt, and tried to relax as we headed towards the city. We had been travelling for some time through the suburbs of Islamabad past a variety of houses, from slums to modest homes and the occasional very large mansion, when we came into an area of rather posh houses with beautiful gardens and immaculately groomed lawns. By then I'd begun to wonder who this Beryl was.

I plucked up courage and asked, 'Beryl, have you lived here long?' just as we turned into the heavily guarded grounds of the British Embassy complex, and she replied that her husband was the British Ambassador! The driver drove off after dropping us outside the imposing residence. As the servants collected my bags, I smiled to myself, completely amazed at the place around me and the fact that I was privileged enough to be staying there – a stark contrast to my tiny tent in Somalia! Guiding me inside, Beryl said, 'Make yourself at home. You may like to take a shower and have a rest. Lunch is at 1.00pm. If you'd like to join us, then just wander down to the dining room. My husband will be home for lunch today and you'll have a chance to meet him.' I was shown to my beautifully furnished room, which was enormous. Looking out the window, I noticed a big, beautiful swimming pool below. It was all very unexpected! Such luxury!

With the door closed, I stretched out on the bed. I hadn't been in such a nice place for a very long time. Marvelling at my coming from a dust-covered weather-beaten tent in Somalia to this luxurious double bed with its clean white sheets made me smile at the odd turns and twists in my life. Conscious of time, I roused myself, showered, and then blissfully slept, first setting my alarm so as not to be late for lunch. I woke up some hours later and wandered down to the dining room. Without really knowing why, I felt extremely nervous. My nervousness soon disappeared at the welcome from Oliver, the British Ambassador, and Beryl, both putting me at ease in this new country. Like so many other things in the residence, the dining table was massive, and as I took my seat, I noticed the number of knives and forks on each side of the place settings. The etiquette lessons we'd been given by the principal's wife at Bible College in Tasmania flashed into my mind: Start at the outside and work your way in. I did just that, and I managed very well. We had a lovely conversation over lunch, and I felt very much at home with my delightful host and hostess in the few days I spent with them in their calm and peaceful surroundings. I wasn't to know it then, but in the days, months and years that followed, Oliver and Beryl were to become like parents; not only to me, but to all the Bannu ladies.

Bannu Beginnings

A few days after my arrival, my hosts arranged for me to be driven to Bannu, an isolated and conservative Muslim frontier city on the border of the tribal area in what was then known as the North-West Frontier Province of Pakistan, over 350 kms from Islamabad. After a long drive on often narrow and dangerous roads, I finally arrived at the Pennell Memorial Hospital. This was a Christian Mission Hospital which was well known for the wonderful care it gave all people who came seeking medical help. There, I joined four English women who had lived in Bannu for several years; two nurses, one doctor, Ruth Coggan, and one teacher who was also a writer. They all had a deep understanding of the local culture and languages, Urdu and Pashtu, and were gifted, not only in their roles in the hospital, but also musically, using their skills to entertain themselves in the evenings. I certainly was the odd one out, having no musical talent whatsoever! Despite this shortcoming of mine, which didn't seem to bother them, they went out of their way to make me feel welcome. They were known collectively as the 'Bannu ladies,' a title given to them by the British Embassy wives who loved to come and visit us in Bannu regularly during the year; I was now one of them.

We lived in the main five-bedroomed house, which had been built for the British Army and later taken over by Dr Theodore Pennell and his mother in the early 1900s. Theodore Pennell was a gifted young doctor who had turned his back on a very promising medical career in England to follow the call of God on his life. Through the Church Mission Society, he came to Bannu in 1893, and went about using his skills to assist the local tribal and Afghan people, dressing like a Pathan (an ethnic Afghan Muslim) and speaking fluent Urdu and Pashtu (Pashtu being the main language of the Afghans in this area of what was then India, later Pakistan).

Not only did Pennell establish the hospital in Bannu, but he also spent time and effort founding schools. Sadly, he died at a young age. In 1912 a very sick patient was admitted to Bannu hospital in a critical condition, requiring surgery. Pennell's colleague operated on him and fell sick himself. Pennell operated on this colleague and he too fell sick. Within a few days, his colleague died, followed three days later by Pennell, of septicaemia, conscious to the end and unafraid of death. He was only in his mid-forties. The deaths of the two doctors left the hospital without one until reinforcements came from Peshawar.

It was as if Doctor Pennell still resided in the house where I was now living. All his furniture, many of his diaries, and a collection of his instruments were still in the building. I enjoyed reading his diaries, which had fascinating descriptions of the planning for the great exodus to the hills in the summer, when the Bannu temperatures could rise to 40°C (In winter the temperatures could drop to 7°C). The diaries recorded how many elephants, how many servants, and what food supplies were needed for the white migration to the hills of Murree. I could sit at his desk and read, and imagine I was planning this adventure with him.

Pennell House, which was to become my home for the next few years, was situated on a large complex with a mud brick wall surrounding it. On the compound were two other houses, the generator shed and an Anglican Church, where a communion service was offered every Sunday by an Anglican padre who lived near the hospital. The services were all in Urdu, but my colleagues did translate the key points of the sermon to me. I enjoyed it when we had visiting clergy, including Ruth's father and mother, Lord Donald, a former Archbishop of Canterbury, and Lady Jean Coggan. His sermon was delivered first in English (this was great for me, and I appreciated what he had to share) then translated into Urdu.

The house where we lived was made from mud brick and was beautifully cool in the hot Bannu summers but freezing cold in the winter. There was a large dining room, and off this room was the sitting room which had a small fireplace. Each bedroom had its own local version of an 'ensuite' which consisted of a cold shower, and a flush toilet. When I first arrived, there was no hot water, and every Sunday night the servant would bring a large container of hot water into our individual bathrooms and pour the water into a small tin bath, which took some skill getting into and even more skill getting out of! The kitchen was in a separate shed near the back door and consisted of very primitive kerosene stoves, with the refrigerator in the dining room. A lovely porch out the back was the meeting place for Earl Grey tea and cake, every afternoon at 4pm. While I was living in Bannu, we got a hot water system installed and a telephone connected, both major events for us all. We had a cook, a gardener and a servant who assisted us inside the house. The house had a large back yard and garden which were cared for by our gardener. We also had an armed guard who was given a few bullets each night to put into his gun. If he didn't use the bullets at night, then his gun was returned to the Pakistani doctor's house across the road from the female hospital, along with the bullets! All in all, it was a busy and pleasant household and lovely retreat from our work.

I had been there a short time when a new nurse named Pauline arrived from England. Her arrival was considered an opportune time to send both of us to a language school in Murree (in the hills above Islamabad, six hours by road from Bannu), where we would start a six-week course in Urdu. It wasn't something that I was looking forward to at all; dyslexic as I was, my history of learning a foreign language was dismal, to put it mildly. On our way there, we happily stayed a few days at the British Embassy in Islamabad, before being chauffeur-driven on to Murree with Oliver, the ambassador, who was to attend the Murree Christian School's production of the musical *Oliver*. Our new accommodation in Murree was a bit of a change of scenery, and the Ambassador was as shocked as we were when he dropped us off. We'd been allocated a tiny room above the language school with two beds and a commode for a toilet, which was emptied by a man three times daily. That was the arrangement, and that's what we had to put up with! We just had to accept it and carry on. Early that evening, the ambassador collected us, and his driver drove us to the school for the evening performance of *Oliver*. (Our arriving with the ambassador led everyone to believe we were his daughters, which we found highly amusing.) It was a fun night; the performance lively and entertaining. After the show we were dropped off at our accommodation with promises from Ambassador Oliver that we would always be welcome at the Embassy. Pauline and I climbed into our beds, hoping to get some sleep before the language school started in the morning.

When we turned up at our new school, the teachers and other students were very surprised to see us there. They had thought we were the ambassador's daughters! By the end of that first day, struggling with my first attempts to learn Urdu, I wished I was the ambassador's daughter; then I could have gone back with him to Islamabad! Attending those language classes was a miserable time for me. As the weeks went by, I struggled more and more with learning how to speak and understand the language, and I wasn't making much progress. Even more challenging was the written script, which was not the Roman script that I was used to and confused me even more!

Barbara Walker

If you don't ask, you won't get!

Our living quarters were hardly ideal, either, although we tried to make the best of it and my time outside of the classroom wasn't much more pleasant than my time in it. However, ever the resourceful Kiwi, I soon found an opportunity for an upgrade of our accommodation. One day, while going for a walk in a direction I hadn't wandered before, I came across a beautiful house. When I asked about it, I was told it belonged to the New Zealand Church Missionary Society (NZCMS). Immediately, my mind began to work overtime. In no time at all, miraculously (through my connections with NZCMS), my friend Pauline and I were able to move into this lovely house! Although I still floundered in my attempts to learn the language, the nicer environment lifted my spirits enormously. As the days went by, Pauline and I became friendly with some Irish Catholic priests who were also learning Urdu. They were lovely guys and we just clicked with them. Some evenings they would come and play cards with us. On odd occasions the ambassador Oliver would be driven up from Islamabad and he would join us for dinner. We were soon very good at playing cards and spent many a night relaxing and laughing. Sadly, very little Urdu was learnt, but I became very good at playing cards.

After the six weeks were up, we headed back to Bannu. My friend Pauline was better at Urdu than I was, and with many of our patients being from Afghanistan, there was a need for other languages as well, particularly Pashto. I knew only a few words of Urdu, and had no other languages, so had to rely on the Pakistani staff who had some English, to be my interpreters. I am forever indebted to my colleagues and to those Pakistani staff members who patiently translated for me during my time in Bannu. We all have talents in different areas. Learning foreign languages is not a talent I have been blessed with, and it was a challenge in my multicultural life. The blessing that came with this was the people who willingly supported me, and it may have been a way of God making me more willing to accept help from others.

30. Midwifery on the Front Line: Extraordinary Circumstances and Extraordinary Measures

Questionable practice

Although there was a Government hospital in Bannu, the reputation of the Pennell Memorial Hospital, and especially the dedication of Dr Ruth, meant that we always had large numbers of patients, especially women, coming to us from Bannu town, the villages nearby, and isolated tribal areas, as well as Afghanistan. Dr Ruth was a very skilled obstetrician and gynaecologist from England who had saved many women's lives in her time and had been working in Bannu for several years before I arrived. Because of my passion for midwifery, I asked if she would teach me all she knew about obstetrics and she did. She was willing to teach me skills that midwives in New Zealand would not ordinarily be taught, and for that I was very grateful. During my years in Bannu, she taught me how to use Neville Barnes, Keillands, and craniotomy forceps, how to master the ventouse vacuum extraction machine and the complicated and very delicate procedure of internal versions and breech extractions. It was fortunate that Dr Ruth had chosen to devote her time and skills to this little corner of the world; they were sorely needed at times, and she, and we, were able to make a difference in the lives of so many there.

In that part of the world, most women were delivered by the traditional birth attendants (TBAs), wise women who had learnt their midwifery skills from their mothers, who had learnt from theirs; knowledge passed down through many generations. Sadly, many of the treatments the TBAs gave the women resulted in serious complications. When things went wrong, as they often did, the women would be brought into our hospital to be treated there by Dr Ruth and us. We always prayed before doing deliveries or operations and thanked God for the safe delivery afterwards; some of the practices of the TBAs put the pregnant woman and her unborn baby at severe risk. For example, one widespread practice was to inject the woman in labour with oxytocin or ergometrine drugs, a drug commonly used to contract the uterus after delivery. Unfortunately, the TBAs would inject the drug pre-delivery, to induce stronger contractions, a practice which often resulted in dead babies, and even in maternal deaths due to ruptured uterus. At times we were able to carry out an emergency hysterectomy; this saved the woman's life but meant she could no longer have children. With such a status, no one would marry her, no one would really want her, and she would became an outcast in society.

Neonatal Tetanus

Another common TBA practice was to cut the baby's cord with a knife – the same knife that may have been used to cut grass; a dangerous practice, to say the least. Over the years, we had several newborns brought into the hospital suffering from tetanus because of this practice, and we had great difficulty nursing these poor wee babies. Despite giving them large doses of Valium, we struggled to get their fitting under control. I still have the heart-wrenching image in my mind of these tiny babies shaking violently, their wee hands tightly clenched. After dealing with several such cases, we needed to take action and set up a vaccination programme in the hospital, encouraging the mothers to come and bring their children to be vaccinated, and pregnant women to come themselves, to have their tetanus injections before they delivered. These mothers valued the immunization programme so highly that they would walk for many miles, often in the heat of the day, to bring their babies to the vaccination clinic at the hospital, accepting whatever help we offered to keep their babies healthy.

Prolapsed cords

Working as a midwife in the area, one never knew what was going to happen next. One day, a woman arrived already in advanced labour. Dr Ruth was in the middle of an operation and was due to be in theatre for an hour or so, so I took this woman into our delivery room. As I was examining her abdomen, her waters broke. Within minutes, we could see there was a prolapsed cord. In any place in the world, this is an emergency, as the blood flow to the baby is compromised and the baby is at risk of dying. In Bannu, it was no different. We got word to Dr Ruth, who said she'd be there as soon as she could. Helped by the Pakistani staff, we managed to get the woman in the correct position (on all fours with her head pointing down onto the bed and her back and backside pointing up into the air). My job was to keep my hand inside her, holding the baby's head up and preventing the cord from being compressed and cutting off the blood supply to the unborn infant. The Pakistani staff gave the patient pain relief and we waited, praying hard for the baby, and the mum. Each time the mother had a contraction, my hand felt as if it was going to be squeezed right off, and after what seemed like a very long time, Dr Ruth arrived. We quickly got the woman onto the trolley, with me holding the unborn baby's head off the still pulsating cord and headed for theatre. The mother was quickly anaesthetised, and Dr Ruth began to perform an emergency Caesarean section. At the right moment, guided by Dr Ruth, I removed my hand and slowly stood up. A minute later, a beautiful baby boy was delivered. His cry brought tears to our eyes. It was such a joy to see this wee baby safe in his mother's arms, and to see the delight on the faces of their family. As a team, we were elated as well.

Blood transfusions

We didn't have the privilege of a blood bank when I was working in Bannu; only a small laboratory, which could do basic tests and crossmatch blood. If a patient came into the hospital and needed a blood transfusion, we would ask the husband or family members to donate blood. If they refused to donate, we were in trouble, and would have to rely on staff to donate, send the family members to the bazaar to buy blood, or somehow manage without. Any visitors who came to visit us (for any reason!) were gently persuaded to donate blood before they left. Many did. Being O Rh negative, the universal donor, I was able to donate blood, and during my five-and-a-half years in Bannu I donated as much as I could. I often used a bit of drama to help to fill our stocks; I would go to the lab and make my donation before going out to the waiting room, an extra-large bandage on my arm, and ask the patient's husband to donate some blood. Very occasionally the husband would do so. But often, the responses from the husbands would range from, 'It will make me weak,' to that of one man who said, 'Let her die. I will get a new wife.' The Pathan men prided themselves on hospitality and bravery but when it came to donating blood, the bravery seemed to be forgotten! I remember two cases where we couldn't get enough blood, and as a result, two women died in front of our eyes. Life was certainly tough for the women of this North-West Frontier Area of Pakistan.

Internal version breech extractions

One day, a woman came into the hospital in strong labour, her unborn baby presenting with a prolapsed arm protruding from the woman's vagina and no foetal heartbeat. We knew that she came from the tribal region of the North-West Frontier Province, bordering Bannu. Because the medical facilities there were severely limited, Dr Ruth was very reluctant to carry out a Caesarean section on this mother, knowing the baby was not alive. Ruth understood that, should the woman become pregnant in the future, the safest place for her to be delivered after already having a Caesarean section would be in a hospital, which were very few and far between in the tribal area. After some discussion, Dr Ruth decided that the safest option for the mother would be to carry out an internal version breech extraction under a spinal anaesthetic. Having seen Dr Ruth complete such a procedure before, I asked if I could do this. She agreed, and after she had given the woman a spinal anaesthetic, I took over and carried out a technique known as an internal version breech extraction, resulting in the delivery of the stillborn baby. Although it was tragic that the baby was a stillborn, it meant that the woman didn't have to undergo a caesarean section for a dead baby. Some years later while working in Zambia, I was able to teach an English doctor at the hospital where I was a nurse midwife the same technique I had learnt from Dr Ruth. This was one of my most memorable maternity cases during my time in Bannu, and it brought back childhood memories of my friend Anne's sheep farm in New Zealand, where her father Clarrie had taught me to do a similar procedure on a pregnant ewe in distress. We all have so much to learn from one another.

Exchange transfusions on new-born babies

Another day at the hospital, a baby was born in serious trouble. Almost before our eyes he was turning yellow, indicating a serious problem with his blood. Dr Ruth and I discussed it and decided that we would carry out a neonatal transfusion. We set up a small area in the delivery room and I donated my O Rh blood for the procedure. Not having an incubator or a paediatrician on hand, we did the best we could in those circumstances; first, we placed the baby on a hot water bottle to regulate his temperature, while continuously monitoring his heart rate with a stethoscope. After praying for divine guidance, Dr Ruth managed to place a thin catheter into the baby's umbilical vein and slowly draw out a small amount of the baby's blood before inserting some of my blood into the infant. We steadily completed the transfusion process, and over the next 24 hours the condition of the baby improved. The improvement continued, and a few days later, the baby and his beaming mother were discharged, much to our delight. Some months afterwards, we were able to do a similar transfusion on another new-born, with another positive result, amazed as always at what we were able to achieve in such simple surroundings, using what we had at hand, and sharing all our resources.

'Call the flying squad!' 'I AM the flying squad!'

During my New Zealand midwifery training, one of the principal texts we used was an excellent book by British midwife Maggie Myles. This was a very practical guide for midwives needing guidance on difficult maternity cases. However, Maggie firmly offered very clear boundaries for midwives who suddenly found themselves facing complex cases outside of their scope of practice; her advice in such situations was to call the 'flying squad.' The 'flying squad' ideally would consist of a team of experienced medical people who could come and assist the midwife or arrange for the pregnant woman to be transferred to hospital, to provide the help that was needed. In Bannu, if Dr Ruth was on duty, she become the key member of our 'flying squad' when a woman in advanced labour arrived at our hospital in a critical condition; a very comforting backup for us all! These women often arrived at our hospital lying in the back of a pickup truck, having travelled from distant tribal areas whose local traditional birth attendants were unable to deliver the mother. If Dr Ruth was out of town, however, it was a very different story.

I found this out one day when Dr Ruth was away and I suddenly had to become the lead member of our 'flying squad,' when an Afghan woman came into the hospital in advanced labour. In those days, of course, there were no such things as scans, and we had no monitors; my skills as a midwife were very much those of palpation of the woman's abdomen and listening to the foetal heart with a foetal stethoscope. I examined this mother internally as well, and it was then that I realised there was something very wrong. The foetal head that was presenting had a huge fontanelle, a sign of the unborn baby being hydrocephalic, a condition in which there is an accumulation of cerebrospinal fluid within the brain, where, in infants, this fluid enlarges the head. I called over two of my fellow midwives and asked them to examine the woman. One was my friend Heather Sims who just happened to be visiting me in Bannu. I had first met Heather at St Helen's in 1974 when we were working as midwives. I said nothing to them until they had examined the woman. They both confirmed what I was thinking. 'We think this baby is hydrocephalic,' they concluded. The woman continued in very strong labour. I knew that something had to be done or she would rupture her uterus, causing the potential for a dead mother as well as a dead baby. What a dilemma!

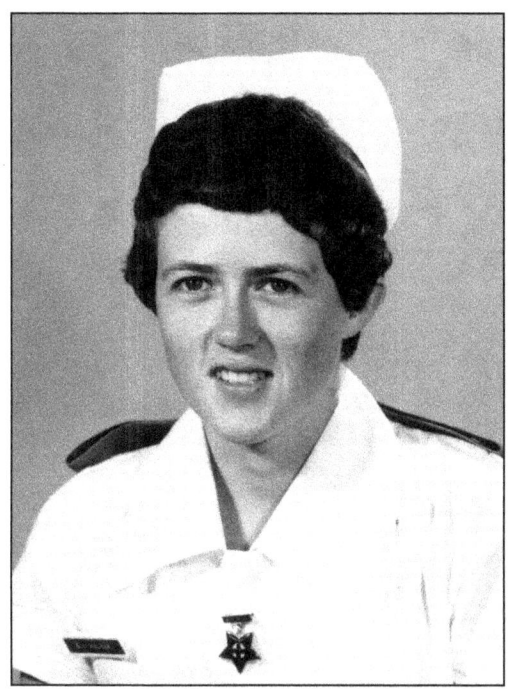

Barbara, Registered Nurse.
Greenlane Hospital, Auckland – 1973.

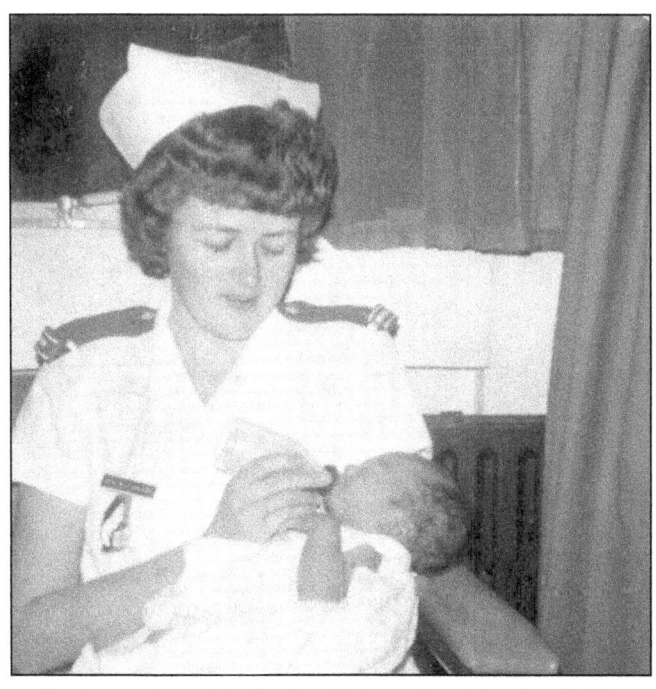

Barbara the midwife. St. Helen's, Auckland – 1974.

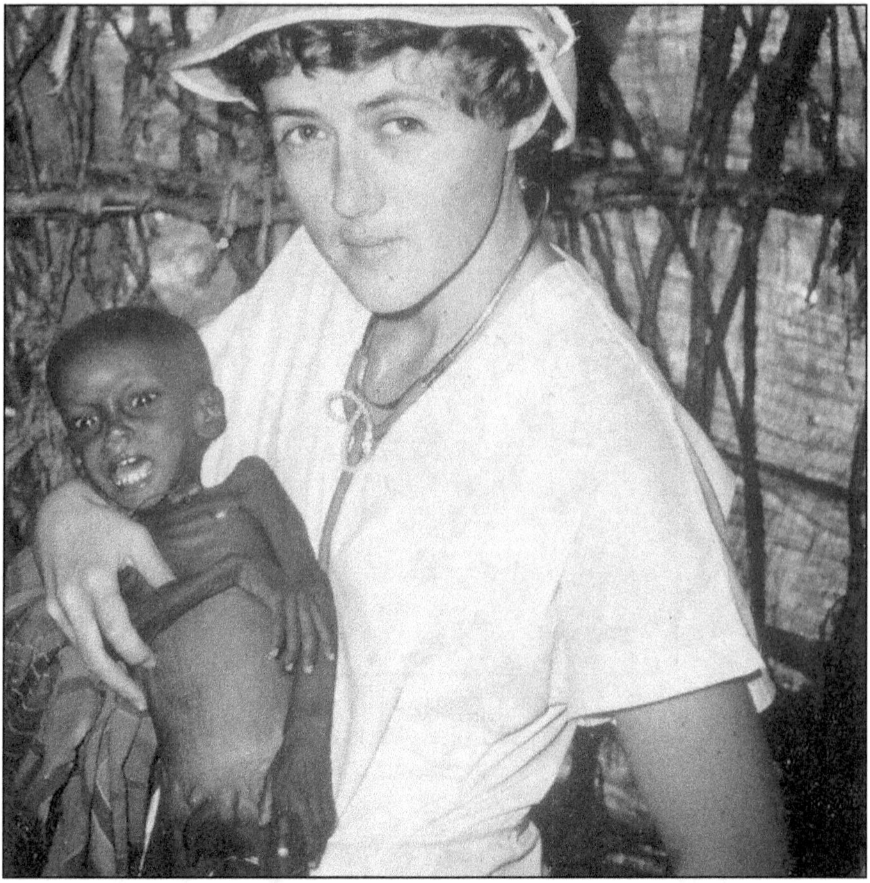

Las Dhure Camp, Somalia – 1980, after being there a number of months. It was tough.

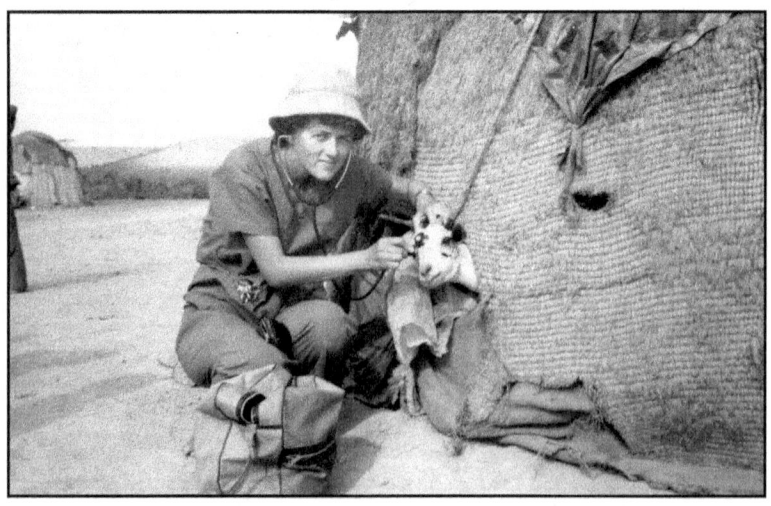

A sense of humour is essential for any aid worker.
Las Dhure Camp, Somalia – 1980.

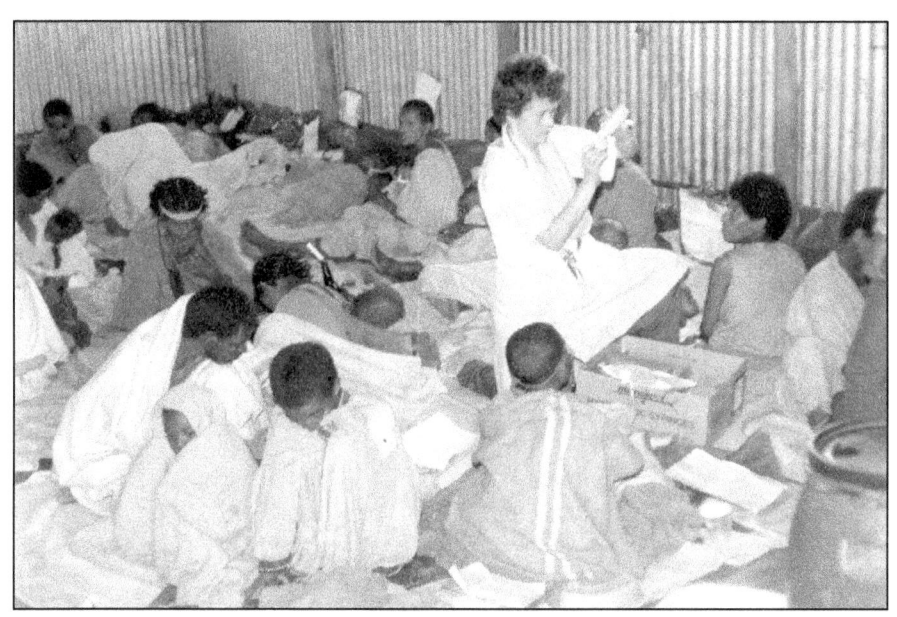

Overcrowded children's ward in Ibnat refugee camp, Ethiopia – 1984.

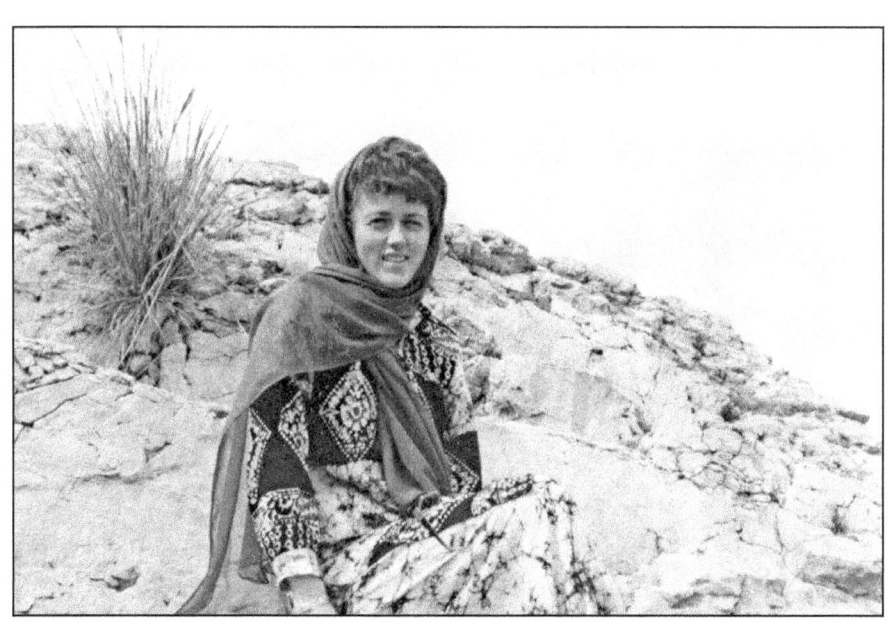

In swimming costume, ready to swim at a dam near the
Pennell Memorial Hospital in Bannu, Pakistan – c.1984.

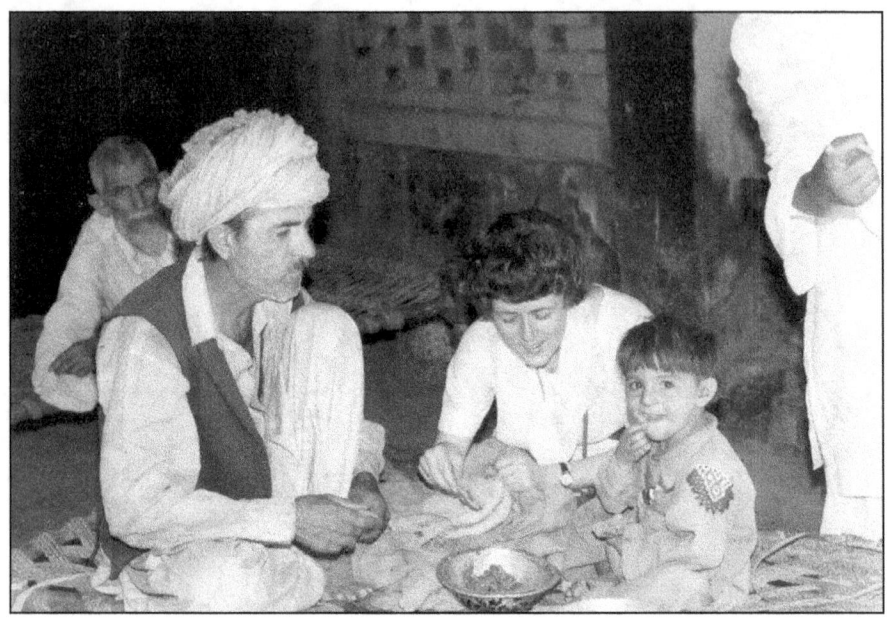

An invitation to join an Afghan family for a meal at the Pennell Memorial Hospital, Bannu, Pakistan – 1985.

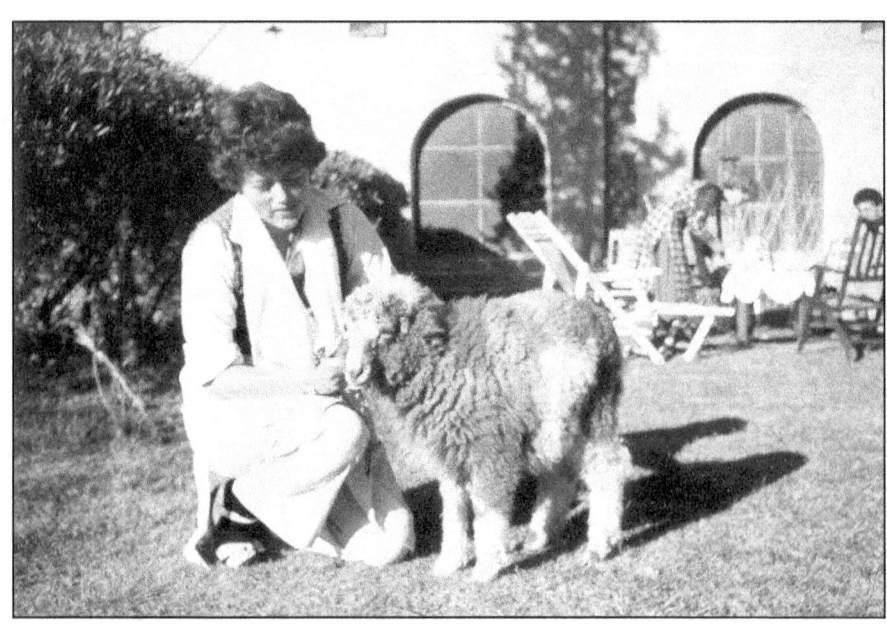

Pet sheep in Bannu, North West Frontier Province, Pakistan – 1986.

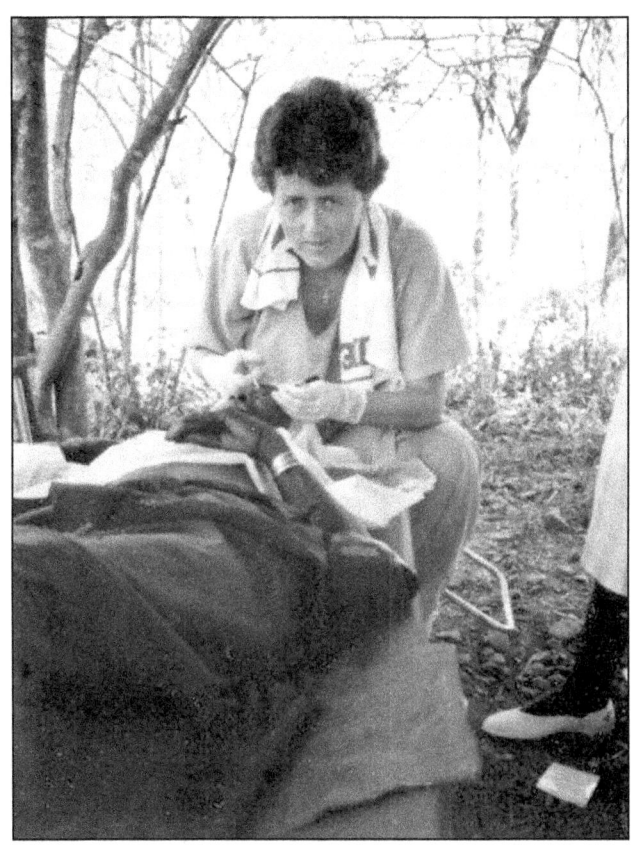

"Eye Surgeon" performing trachoma operations in a remote village in Northern Kenya – 1988.

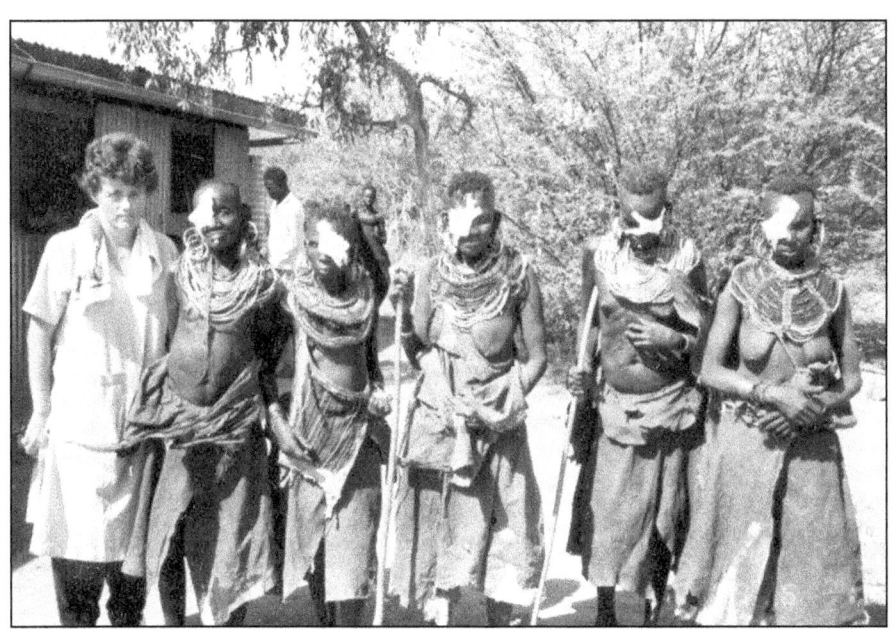

A morning clinic, after eye surgery in a remote village in Northern Kenya – 1988.

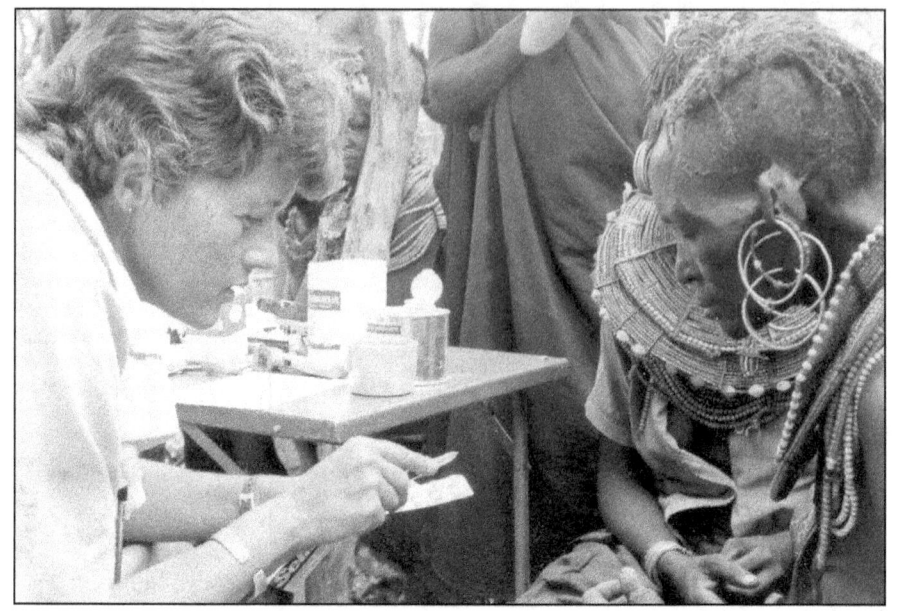

With Pokot women in Northern Kenya – 1988.

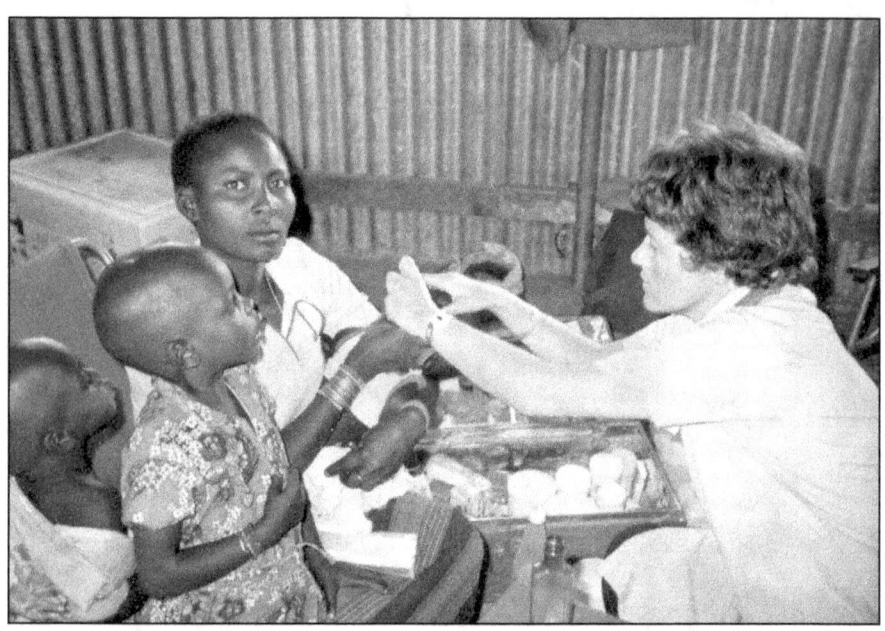

Outpatient Clinic in a remote Northern Kenyan village – 1989.

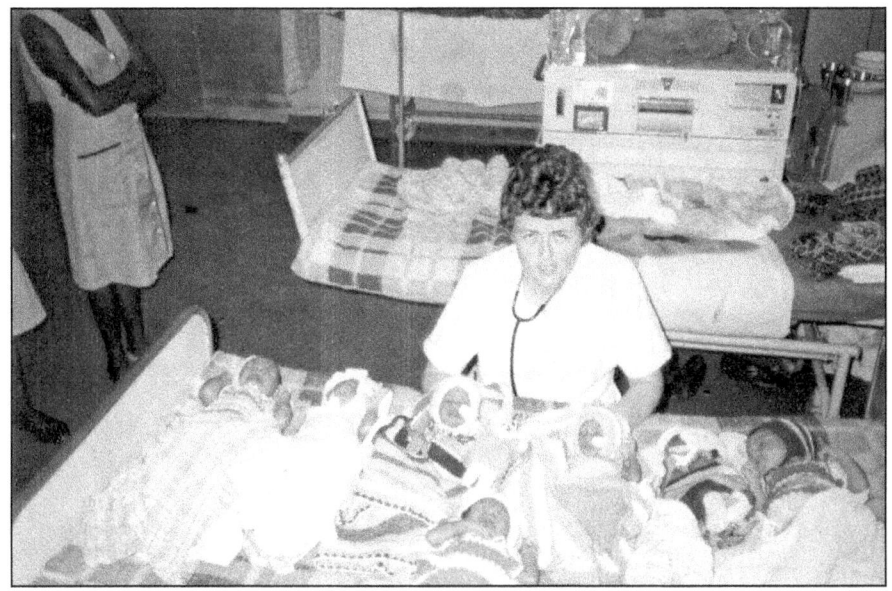

A collection of sets of twins Barbara was involved in delivering, in Mpongwe, Zambia – 1990.

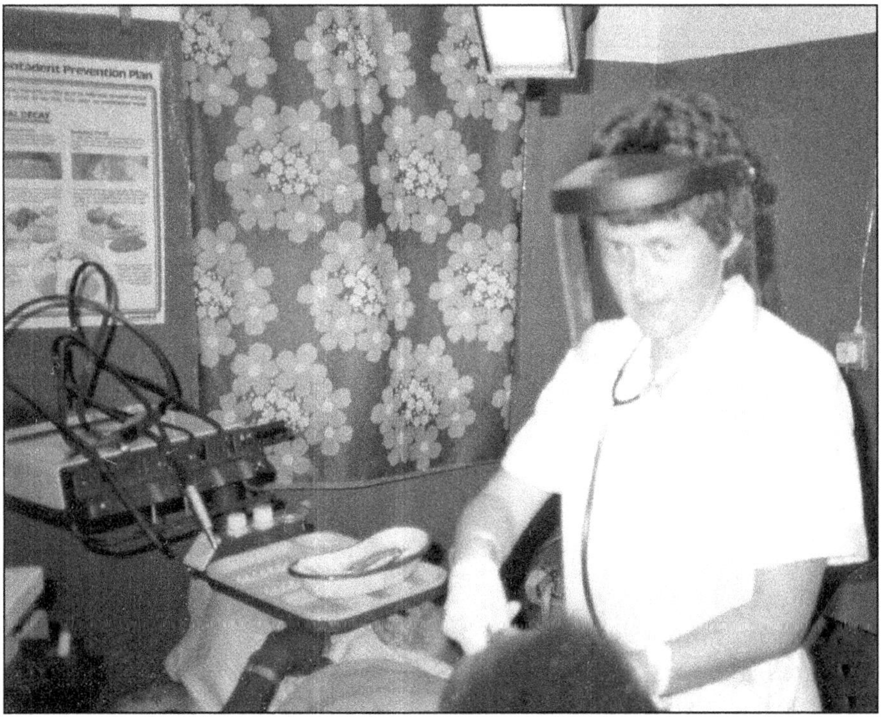

"Dentist" Barbara at Mpongwe Mission Hospital, Zambia – 1991.

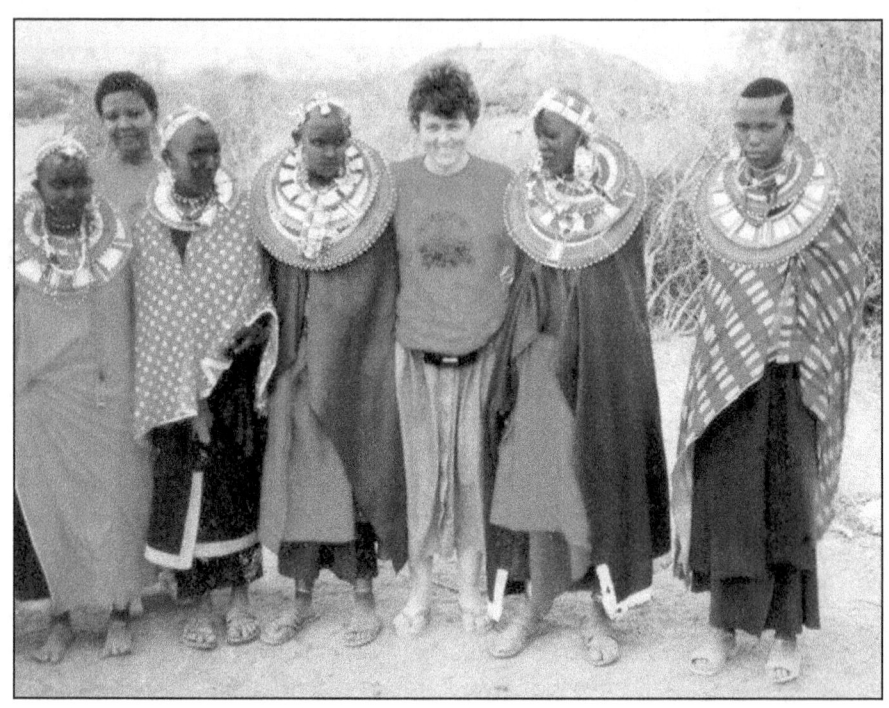

Barbara's Masai friends, with interpreter Ruth, in Tanzania – 1995.

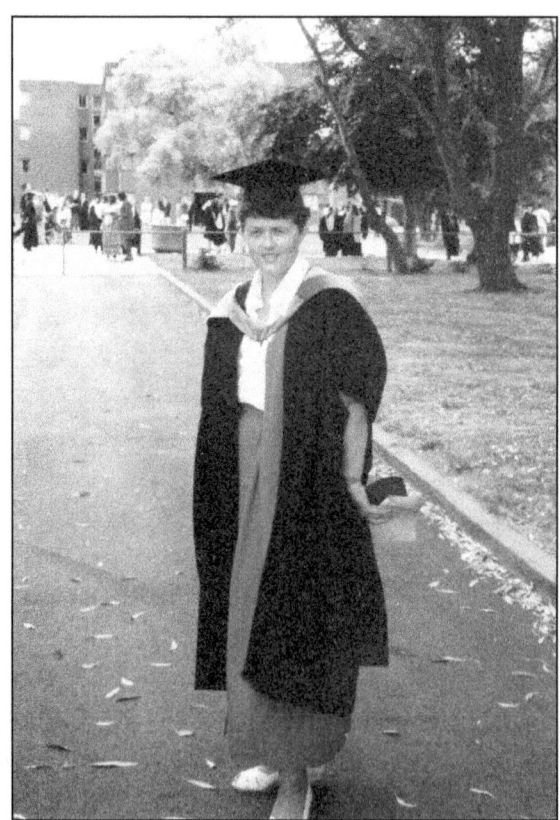

Barbara MSc in Medical Anthropology, graduation day, Brunel University, London – 1995.

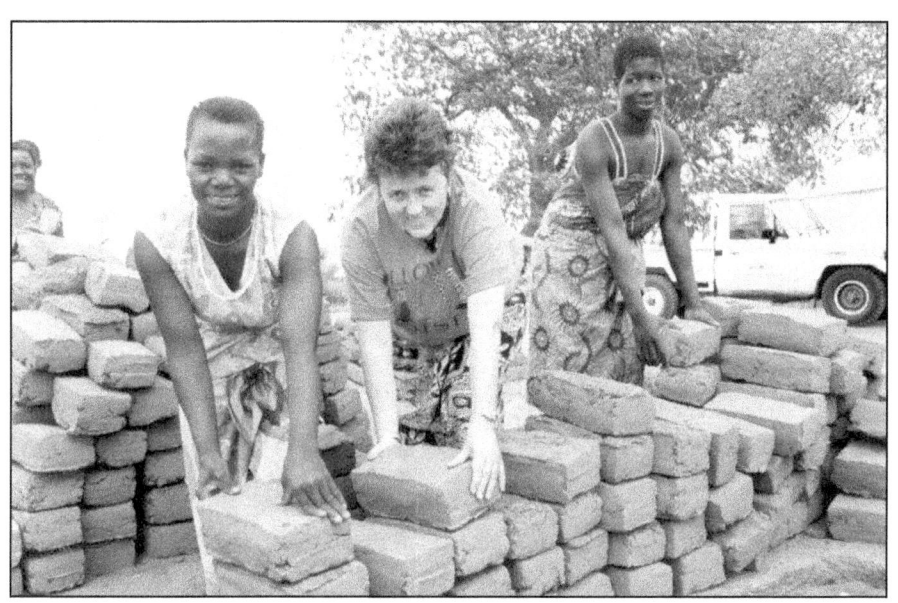

Barbara and local women making mud bricks to be used for building local houses, in Mozambique – 1996

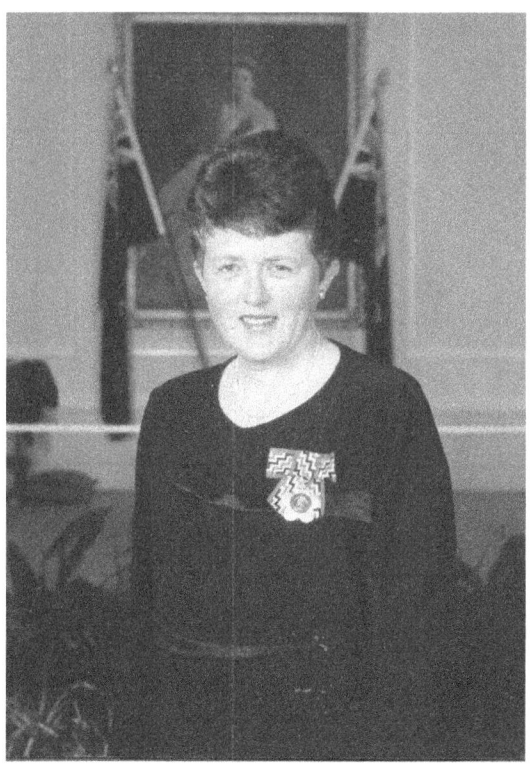

Barbara awarded the QSO – Queens Service Order – for her work overseas and in the Hokianga in Northland – 2000.
(Photo by Woolf Photography, Wellington.)

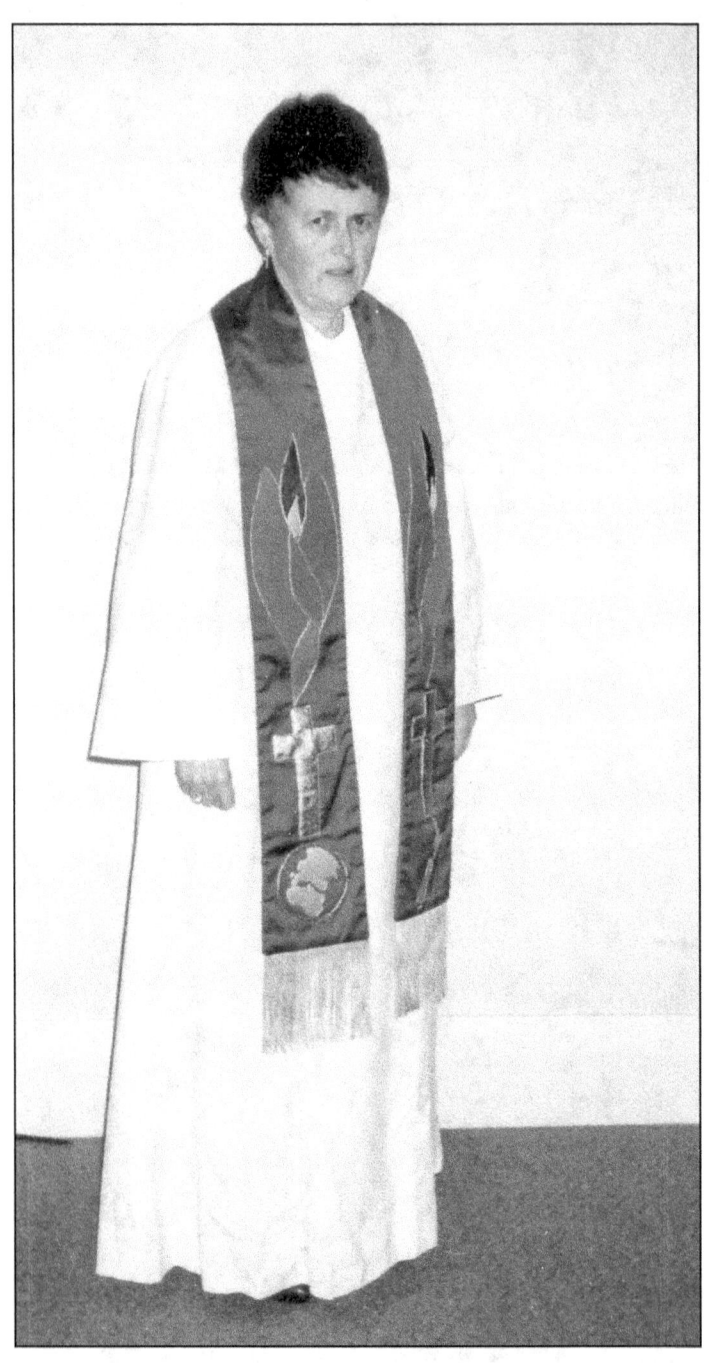
Rev Barbara Walker, Ordained Anglican Priest, Dunedin – 2004.

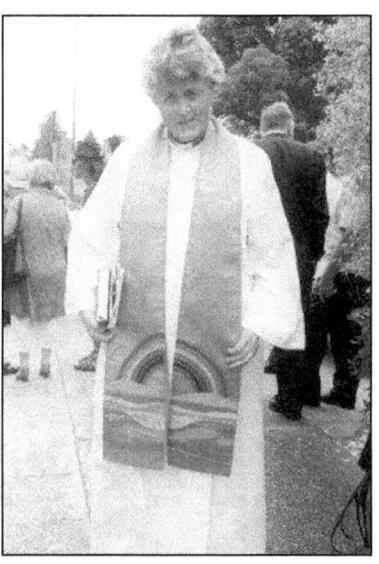

Barbara officiating at her Dad's funeral in Whakatane – 2010.

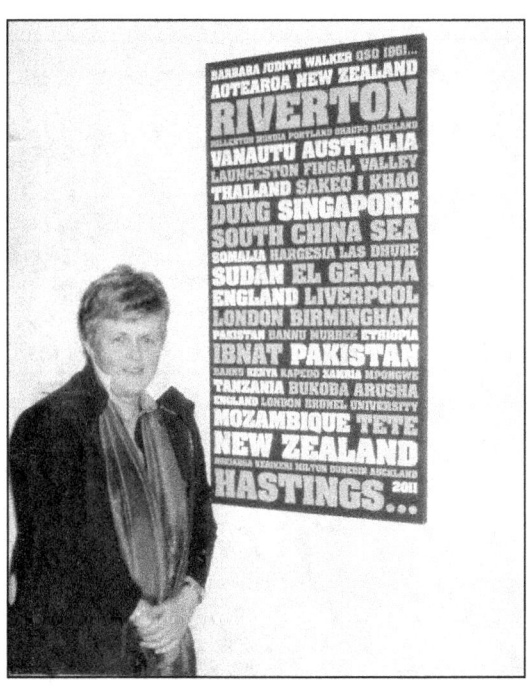

Barb's life journey and the places she has lived and worked in – 2011.

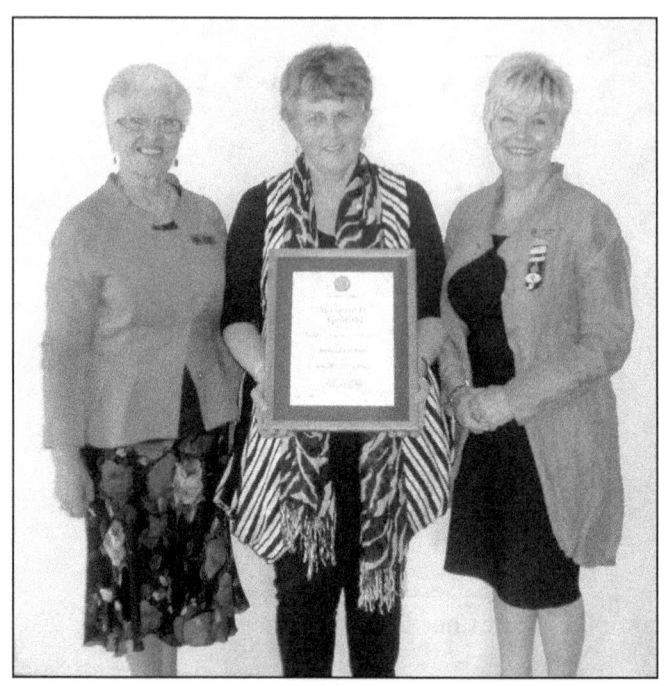

Barbara receiving The International Margarette Golding Award – 2012.

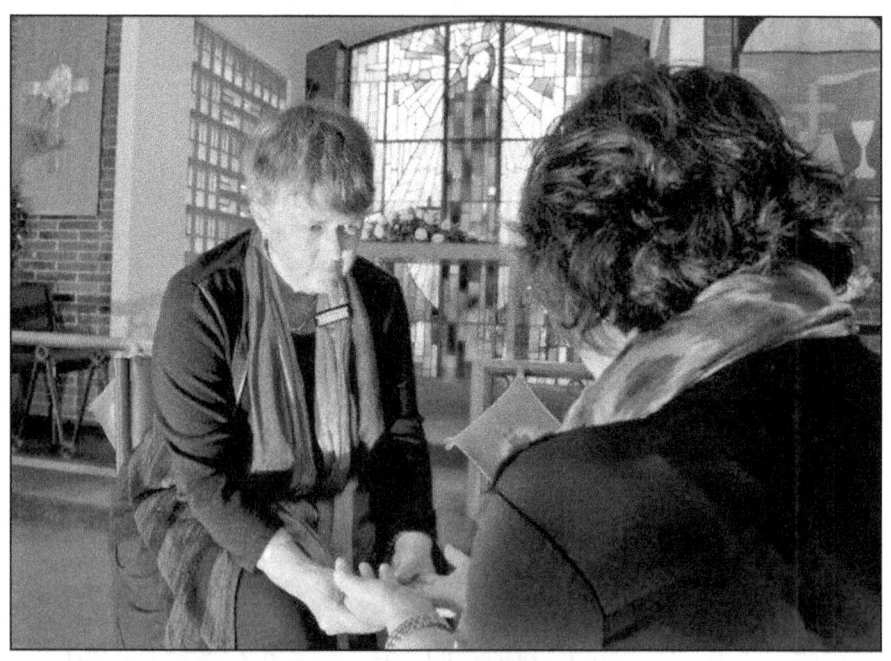

Barbara, hospital chaplain at
Hawkes Bay Fallen Soldiers' Memorial Hospital, Hastings – 2019.

How I wished Dr Ruth had been there! But she wasn't. So, remembering what she had shown me, and explaining to the mother through one of the local staff what was happening and that her baby was not going to be born alive, we prayed. Then I prepared myself to perform my first craniotomy. I inserted the special forceps, piercing the baby's fontanelle. Suddenly, an enormous shower of fluid flowed out. It poured out into a large stainless-steel bucket, and within moments the bucket was full to overflowing. I looked at my colleague, relieved but also saddened. I had saved the mother's life, but the baby had died. Very soon after that, the woman gave a determined push and the baby was delivered; a little boy, dead.

At the end of the day as I reflected on this delivery, I had very mixed emotions; I had saved the mother but, in order to do so, I had to sacrifice the baby. Had I made the right decision? If I had done nothing, then both the mother and her unborn baby would have died; by carrying out the procedure, at least the mother had lived.

This case illustrates how working in such isolated places is tough sometimes, and professionals often must make life and death decisions. To this day, I believe it was the only choice I had, and I am grateful to the other midwives who agreed with my original diagnosis. No amount of experience can ever harden the human heart to situations like that one, and time doesn't always fade the memories.

The building of a new midwifery unit

Our small delivery room was very basic and not suitable for the more complex obstetrics procedures we were performing daily. We had many discussions about the need to build a new one. Our team of expats had recently expanded with the addition of an Aussie nurse, Rosemary Holt, who happened to have contacts in Australia with the potential to help fund some of the cost of building a desperately needed unit. Over the next year or so, funding came through from various sources around the world, including a large gift from the Anglican Archbishop of Sydney's fund. Plans were drawn up, and the building of the unit began. When the very modest new midwifery unit opened, it was a special day for us. It was also a proud day for all the women of the area, and celebrations included traditional dancing, food, speeches and prayer. This spacious, modern, two-roomed midwifery unit was a 100% improvement on the tiny room we had used previously and meant that we could have two women delivering at the same time on our two very modern delivery beds.

Many women arrived at the hospital in an advanced stage of labour, having experienced serious complications in their home villages. They often came from areas in the tribal area of Pakistan and many were Afghan refugees. Because of our facilities, equipment and skills, we were able to save the lives of hundreds of these mothers and their babies, and we were grateful for the support our work received from different groups all over the world, who enabled us to do so.

31. Life in Bannu

Originally, I had the intention of going to Bannu for two years, but I ended up staying there for more than five. I loved the extremely challenging obstetrics and working alongside Dr Ruth and my work colleagues, but I struggled living in the very restricted society which was Bannu in the 1980s. One example of the restrictions was the way that the hospital had a number of wards for female patients on one side of the road, with male patients on the other side. This could make things challenging. We expat nurses were able to work on both sides, and I would go over to the male hospital to do a ward round with the Pakistani Doctor a couple of days a week, but the Pakistani nurses were assigned to either the female or male side, depending on their gender, (though our Pakistani staff who assisted in our operating theatre were both female and male). The segregation wasn't just during work; after hours, we were essentially confined to the compound of the hospital and strongly discouraged from going outside it for things like shopping. Bannu was a very conservative Muslim city where local women were very rarely seen in public, and if they were, they would be totally covered by their burkas. On the very odd occasions that we did go into the shopping area, we had our heads covered and wore shalwar kameez. However, we were able to leave the compound when we were invited to weddings, which was often, and these were very different to New Zealand weddings. During the celebration, female guests would remain in one part of the house and male guests in another, and never the twain would meet. The Bannu Ladies were always served the wedding food in a separate room and were treated like VIPs. One highlight of being invited to a wedding meant that we were able to get new shalwar kameez, along with dupattas, and the female staff were able to give us advice on what the latest fashion was from their relatives in other parts of Pakistan, like Lahore or Islamabad. We enjoyed being welcomed into the community this way and being able to learn about such a different culture from our own.

We were occasionally able to take advantage of our awareness of the local traditions though. During the annual Muslim festival of Ramadan we, the Bannu Ladies, were permitted go for an early evening bike ride around the area where we lived, known as the cantonment area, as this was where the local military residential accommodation was located. We could venture on our bikes at this time as the local Muslim community would be inside their houses breaking their fast. This short taste of freedom would last for little more than 30 minutes and was the only time we were all able to ride our bikes around the cantonment area enjoying the simple freedom we all took for granted in our own worlds.

On rare occasions one of the local business men, who was a very good friend of our hospital's Pakistani doctor, would come and offer to take us up to the nearby dam for a swim and a cup of tea in the segregated refreshment area in the dam's small tea house. Whenever he offered me the keys, I would take up his offer and drive us Bannu Ladies to the dam for a swim, one of the few things I could do which felt like normality for me in this very strict society.

When we did go for a swim, we didn't wear togs, but our Pakistani clothes, and yes, we had our heads covered when we swam. It was like being on show, as several local men would watch us swimming in the dam while their wives and children were in seclusion inside the tea house. Times like those made me feel very far from home. Maybe even more so because such a social life was so limited, but I loved the work in the hospital and that became my focus. At times, I suspect I became a workaholic. I can see now that this helped me to survive.

In 1983, as the first New Zealander ever to work in Bannu, I found it hard to settle into the formal setting. At that time, Russia had invaded Afghanistan in the north and millions of refugees were pouring across the border into Pakistan, mainly into Peshawar, the nearest big city. America was supporting the Mujahideen, a large group of well-equipped and trained fighters who were based in Pakistan who carried out raids into Afghanistan. (The Taliban movement hadn't been formed at that time.) It was a dangerous time and place, and I often felt very far away from friends and family.

32. Interlude: from Bannu to Ethiopia

One day in 1985, I received a request from World Vision, asking if I would be willing to go to Ethiopia to help in the unfolding famine crisis. The cry for experienced relief and disaster medical staff had gone out around the world, and New Zealanders were among the many who responded. At the time, Dr Ruth was about to have a brief break in England, and I knew that the local government hospital in Bannu, although the second choice for many patients, would cope with any complicated maternity cases. The timing seemed right for me to go to Ethiopia and my colleagues agreed. I contacted World Vision and flew to Ethiopia to assist in the ongoing disaster there, opening yet another new chapter in my life.

Ethiopia: First impressions

I wasn't quite sure what to expect on arrival in Ibnat. Ethiopia was experiencing a severe drought throughout a vast area of the country, which had begun in 1983. By early 1985, the situation was dire, and thousands of Ethiopians had become refugees in their own country. Finally, to relieve the situation, the government had set up camps in various areas, including the remote settlement of Ibnat, a small town on a sparsely treed, dust-bowl plateau in the western Gondar region of Africa's Great Rift Valley. Winds continually swept along its plains, creating dust storms and coating everything in their thick grit. The occasional shower of rain turned the dust into sticky clay mud that stuck to shoes like porridge. It wasn't a welcoming or enticing environment, but it was a politically neutral area, and as the place chosen by the government to set up refuge, it was the only hope for many.

Hoping to find food and shelter, famine victims trekked towards the camps with nothing but the clothes on their backs. Many died en-route from sickness and malnutrition, leaving hundreds of unaccompanied elders and orphans to make their way to these makeshift shelters. By early 1985, Ibnat was swollen with a floodtide of such displaced people, with more arriving each day. Chaos reigned as Ethiopian military officials struggled to cope with the influx. The worst-affected people were nomadic pastoralists from the Wollo, Tigre, and Gondar regions whose herds and flocks had died of starvation as grasslands gradually became deserts. As a newcomer, I was told that Ethiopia's Marxist government of the time despised the Wollo people, who were seen by officials as a major burden; a group that was assumed to be uneducated and lower caste. Consequently, to stop the Wollos from reaching the camps, government officials tried to block them at mountain passes and on dry riverbeds. Nevertheless, thousands of these nomadic people managed to reach Ibnat and other camps located in the region. Although there was no official census, estimates of the number of people streaming into Ibnat ranged from 55,000 to 80,000, the population of a typical small town.

Infrastructure, shelter, food, water and medical care were basic requirements, and providing these quickly and effectively was a challenge. Sourcing aid workers to do so was vital. There was international awareness of the plight of Ethiopia at the time, and multiple groups had committed to help. By April, World Vision International had mobilised an international medical team to staff a tent 'hospital' and feeding centres, set up in Ibnat by World Vision Ethiopia. Other international aid agencies were arriving in other parts of Ethiopia to help as well.

In May, I left Pakistan and flew to Addis Ababa, Ethiopia's capital city, and then on to Ibnat in a World Vision 19-seat Twin Otter plane. After a three-hour flight from Addis, the plane prepared to land on Ibnat's grassy airstrip. Through the cabin window, I could see acres of hastily erected huts which were made from the UNHCR plastic sheeting, some with grassed roofs. These huts were placed row upon row in the barren, dry land. Suddenly the reality hit me; this desolate place was to be my home for the next six months. When I disembarked, a World Vision colleague in a dusty Land Cruiser was waiting to meet me.

As we drove along the dirt road running between the camp and the World Vision site, my colleague pointed out the tent 'hospital,' which I would soon learn consisted of several large canvas tents and a few smaller ones. In each 'ward,' patients lay on plastic sheeting placed over a dirt floor. There were no beds, mattresses, sheets or pillows, and not enough blankets. Nurses spent hours struggling to insert life-saving drip lines into the veins of emaciated and dehydrated patients. The tent sides didn't reach the ground, and wind often whipped up the sides, pulling out drip lines attached to the walls. We would fight a cholera epidemic and more under these difficult circumstances, accepting what we couldn't change, and doing our best to adapt and meet the needs of our patients.

As for our living conditions, World Vision staff slept in small rooms in a row of corrugated iron huts in a compound not far from the hospital. I shared a room with a fellow Kiwi nurse Carolyn Kippenberger (Kipp), who showed me the ropes in those early days. Our room had a concrete floor and two single beds, but no bathroom, electricity or running water. Our pit latrines, or 'long drop toilets,' were situated 100 metres away in small, corrugated iron shacks with dirt floors. While this accommodation had its challenges, it was the camp itself which proved to be an exceedingly stressful environment; the political situation was tense and there was a constant, heavy presence of military police and soldiers. Ethiopia's Marxist Government didn't really want relief agencies' personnel working in the camps or in our makeshift hospital, but they did want the benefits of food, medical supplies, trucks, radios and blankets that came with us. It was a volatile mix.

The political manoeuvring involved in getting more doctors was soul-destroying. By lobbying officialdom and cutting through red tape, we managed to import some desperately needed medical people, but many who had been granted visas to Ethiopia were refused a permit to the camp and had to fly back to their homelands. At times even we weren't permitted to set foot in the camp and were restricted to the hospital only.

We chafed at these restrictions, knowing there were many seriously ill people on site. We had no choice but to abide by the rules and regulations received from Government officials; failure to do so could mean being asked to leave the country. Our international team included nurses, engineers, administrators and practical New Zealanders who were always willing to roll up their shirtsleeves and work. We were assisted by local Ethiopian workers, including nurses, a few doctors, engineers, guards and kitchen staff who catered for us and our many visitors. World Vision International was working in partnership with other agencies elsewhere in Ethiopia during this time, as the scale of the disaster was too big for one aid agency. Irish Concern and Save the Children were two such agencies working with us at Ibnat. We tried to ignore the politics; we had enough to focus on with the challenges involved in running such a place.

Everyday life in the camp

One of the most pressing necessities for everyone at the camp was water, which was scarce and therefore precious. Initially when the camp was set up, aid workers were restricted to three litres of boiled water per day, and supplies were limited. By the time I arrived, water was being trucked into the camp regularly, which helped, but despite being told it was safe, we continued to boil it. Fortunately, soon after I arrived, a World Vision America engineer, working with local staff, managed to locate an underground water table and tap into a source of clean drinking water. Pipes with taps attached to large containers were placed strategically around the hospital compound, giving us relatively easy access to water. These water teams worked hard to ensure we had a continuing supply, meanwhile digging hundreds of pit latrines and maintaining the hospital generators. The work to keep the basics available to all at the camp went on round the clock, and every worker we had, not just medical staff, was vital. To have willing volunteers turned away by the very government of the country was frustrating at the best of times, and heart breaking at others. Providing decent refuge for these displaced people just wasn't a priority for the government of the time.

A few weeks before I arrived at Ibnat, the government had burnt the camp down to force people to leave. Seeing clouds of black smoke, my colleagues had rushed over and warned people to leave. Refugees fled as the flames spread, but many were old, blind, deaf, young, sick or physically incapacitated and not everyone managed to escape. No one knows how many refugees died. There was a veil of silence. It was unwise to speak about what had happened. We were guests of the Ethiopian government and warned to be careful about what we said and to whom; commenting on the fire could jeopardise our entire relief operation. As a result of the fire, thousands of refugees fled to the hills, fending for themselves with no sanitation or water, and little food. A few weeks later, people were permitted to return to the soot-charred camp. Refugees slowly trickled back and began to rebuild their huts with sticks, cardboard boxes and UNHCR green plastic sheets; anything that came to hand. In the aftermath, the hospital had an influx of people with cholera and serious chest infections stretching our already over-taxed resources. I had arrived just as the cholera was taking hold.

As well as fighting illness, the famine victims in Ibnat were trying to survive on the meagre rations and contaminated water distributed by government camp officials. Hunger and disease were rife, and the death toll was high. An area outside the camp was designated for burials, but the ground was hard and grave diggers struggled to dig holes, so bodies began to pile up. Often, they were buried in shallow unmarked mass graves. Occasionally a deluge of rain would wash the soil away, exposing decomposing bodies, and raising the risk of infection and contamination of nearby water sources. A related horror was the packs of wild dogs, as big as wolves, which would come down from the hills at night, howling and scavenging for food. These dogs posed a threat to the living and to the dead; we all knew what those dogs were eating.

However, we were there to serve the living, and to do our work the best we could, regardless of the conditions around us. We were medical professionals first and foremost and administering to the famine victims was our focus. The children were the hardest, as many were severely malnourished. We regularly weighed and monitored them and found that many of the children under five weighed less than 45% of their ideal body weight. The children in this state were fed six times a day in the paediatric ward and in feeding centres established near the outpatient clinics, which consisted of numerous poles placed in a large square and covered with a plastic roof.

Every day, staff lit campfires and cooked and served high protein porridge and powdered milk drinks to severely malnourished children. These children were identified by a wrist bracelet and, when a child died, a parent would quickly remove the band and place it on a sibling's wrist to ensure that child would become part of the feeding programme, such was their desperation. These malnourished children were prone to pneumonia, typhoid, cholera, diarrhoea, malaria, relapsing fever and many other unidentified illnesses. They were also riddled with intestinal worms and on admission to the ward, we routinely dosed them with worming medicine. Lifting their blankets in the morning and seeing small piles of wriggling white worms mixed with faeces was an extremely unpleasant sight.

Eventually, these facilities had some improvements when part of our canvas 'hospital' was replaced by corrugated iron buildings with concrete floors. Patients then slept on plastic sheeting on one-metre square platforms constructed to keep them off the floor, with old blankets and cloths providing some measure of comfort. When I wasn't managing the hospital, I worked on these wards, delivering babies, nursing sick children and operating on patients with trachoma. Fortunately, I had learnt to carry out this trachoma operation in Somalia, under the guidance of a visiting British eye specialist. Disease was an ever-present threat and during my six months at Ibnat, we dealt with several epidemics – measles, typhoid, cholera and relapsing fever – and illnesses like pneumonia, malaria and chronic diarrhoea were common.

Our staff was not immune, and many expatriates contracted a mystery illness which we dubbed 'Ibnat flu.' Symptoms included aching joints and violent chills alternating with raging fevers and hallucinations. Many team members were evacuated to Nairobi Hospital and placed in isolation. Tropical disease experts couldn't identify this frightening illness, but fortunately everyone recovered and returned to Ibnat, or headed home if their contract had finished.

All of us had to be adaptable. Along with my work in the hospital, I held the role of technical manager. This job included organising for a trucking company to come from Gondar, the nearest city, to pump out the hundreds of pit latrines. At the end of my first day in this role, the company boss asked me, 'Where do you want us to dump the sewage?' Dumbfounded, I muttered, 'I don't know!' I hadn't imagined the contract wouldn't include the disposal of the sewage! I talked to camp authorities who suggested dumping the waste material in a remote area of the camp. We learned quickly to make our own decisions in this poorly organised place.

As technical manager, my role encompassed a wide range of hospital management and administration tasks (not including information technology as we didn't have cell phones or the internet in those days). I was wonderfully supported by an Ethiopian administrator, along with expat and Ethiopian colleagues. Much of my time was spent in management; ordering medical supplies and overseeing staff at our very overcrowded 'hospital' and numerous outpatient clinics. One of my other daily chores was to ensure the grass runway was dry enough for the frequent World Vision planes to land; if the tyres on a fully loaded plane got stuck in a boggy patch as it came into land, it could have caused disastrous results for all on board. So, every morning and afternoon I would drive up and down the airstrip to see how far the Land Cruiser tyres sank into the ground. If the ground was too wet, I would radio World Vision in Addis and cancel any scheduled landings. If the ground was dry, I would tell them it was okay to send a plane. This daily decision weighed heavily on me, as cancelling flights meant delays in getting urgently needed medicines and intravenous fluids. Also, staff who'd been having a break in Addis wouldn't be able to return, and others needing a break wouldn't be able to leave. One day, we heard that a massive special transport plane would be making a blanket drop on the airstrip. This was exciting news, as famine refugees were chronically short of blankets. The pilot planned to fly low over the runway and drop 10,000 grey woollen blankets packed in wooden pallets. Unfortunately, many of the pallets broke on landing and blankets were strewn from one end of the runway to the other, meaning we spent hours gathering them up. During a previous air drop in another refugee camp not far from us, a refugee had been killed when he tried to catch a sack of falling maize.

We also had supplies coming in by truck and during my time in Ibnat, the New Zealand Meat Board donated 1,000 tons of lamb chops to World Vision Ethiopia for famine relief. These succulent, delicious brine-cured lamb chops were packed into large plastic buckets (which families later used to carry water and belongings; nothing is wasted in a refugee camp). We distributed the lamb chops among the 100 or so children and their accompanying parents or caregivers in the paediatric ward. The lamb chops were boiled in massive pots on wooden fires in a make-shift kitchen near the paediatric ward. As we walked down the ward handing out chops, it was heart-wrenching to see skeletal hands reaching out from under blankets to grasp a chop. Children sucked on the bones for hours, some still clutching them the following day. Kipp and I were thrilled when the lamb chops arrived, as it was a little part of New Zealand coming to this place of suffering and frequent sadness and it certainly brought smiles to the recipients' faces, and to ours. Years later, when speaking at meetings around New Zealand, I met farmers who had donated lambs for the project and others who had organised transportation to Ethiopia. I was personally able to thank these people and tell them what joy those chops had brought to emaciated children.

Politics in the field

Meanwhile, drought conditions were worsening throughout Ethiopia and United Nations officials decided to do a survey of people living in remote areas to try and gauge how big the problem was. They also wanted to know how many potential famine victims were struggling out in the more remote regions, where the famine had truly taken hold. I volunteered to be a data collector and, with two Ethiopian colleagues, boarded a helicopter flown by an Australian pilot. As we flew into the mountains, we were able to view the rugged terrain below through the glass-bottomed helicopter. Landing on rocky patches on mountain tops, we walked to nearby villages. As we approached, children screamed with fear and hid; many had never seen a helicopter, let alone a white person. We gave the villagers high protein biscuits to eat as they shared harrowing stories with my Ethiopian colleagues of the hardships they were facing due to the prolonged drought spreading across the region. We saw many malnourished and infection-prone children and parents said many more had already died. Wherever we landed, people told us the same stories. We encouraged them to leave their homes and come to the camps where they would receive rations and medical care, but most were reluctant to leave their ancestral land and make the long trek to any of the refugee camps within the drought regions. We flew back to Ibnat and discussed the situation with United Nations personnel, who in turn discussed the findings with the officials in the capital, and plans were made as to how to assist the growing number of refugees needing help. There were no simple solutions.

Because of the political situation, we weren't in regular communication with the government for guidance, but with our own agencies and the United Nations. We communicated regularly with the World Vision office in Addis via a two-way radio link and sent reports and letters in a special mail bag on the World Vision plane, which flew to Ibnat regularly, weather permitting. We also had radio contact with the United Nations office in Addis, which was monitoring the refugee situation closely. When a crisis loomed, we would radio a pre-arranged password and UN personnel would fly to the camp to negotiate with the government military overseers. The world's press was roundly condemning the government's inhumane treatment of its own displaced people and, as news spread, supplies began to flood in, but we still were struggling to get experienced medical professionals, who were regularly spending days waiting in Addis for permission to come to Ibnat. The management and administration of the camp was a daily struggle.

The world was paying more attention to Ethiopia than to previous humanitarian crises, in part because of famous and well-off people taking notice and spreading the word; pop singers, movie stars and VIPS often came to visit. They would fly into Ibnat, walk around the camp, ask a few questions, often with a camera crew in tow, and leave. Having worked in several such relief situations, I often struggled with the celebrities, whose approach could appear self-serving and seem like a way of getting personal publicity, but there were some who really wanted to help in whatever way they could. The humanitarian efforts of celebrities like Bono, whom I had the privilege of meeting during my time in Ibnat, Bob Geldof and others helped enormously in raising awareness of the refugees' plight. Band Aid and Live Aid concerts, two such initiatives, were broadcast to 165 countries, raising more than $US150 million for famine relief in Ethiopia, while increasing consciousness around the world.

All the goodwill in the world wasn't stopping the numbers of refugees increasing, however. Camp numbers continued to rise as word got out to refugees elsewhere that food and shelter was available in Ibnat. Deciding there were too many people in the camp there, the government resolved to return some of them to the drought-stricken areas they'd arrived from, often insisting that these areas were slowly coming out of the drought conditions. Tensions mounted as UN officials insisted that the refugees weren't well enough to send home. At one of many related meetings, I challenged an Ethiopian government official and my comments were reported in the British newspaper, *The Guardian*, but thankfully my name wasn't mentioned.

Amidst these tensions, Kipp and I woke one night to the sound of shouts and donkeys braying. The camp was out of bounds to us at night, meaning we couldn't investigate the commotion. Soon afterwards, 220 refugees were found sheltering in an old quarry 20 miles away, having apparently been forced out of the camp at night. Some of the children were at death's door and wearing our feeding centre wrist bands, which identified them as severely malnourished. I radioed United Nations personnel in Addis and they flew in and had in-depth conversations with government and health care officials, and with us. As a result, this group of refugees was returned to the camp and the sick received much-needed food and medical treatment.

These politically charged discussions were stressful, as we didn't know what the government might do next or how we ought to respond. Eventually, it was agreed that some refugees would be trucked back to their homes, but only those strong enough to make the trip. They would be given food rations, plastic sheeting for shelter, some seeds and a hoe so they could dig gardens. They would also be vaccinated against measles and meningitis, two of the major health risks. The day came for many refugees to return to their homelands and, although we had mixed feelings, we had to be cautious about airing our opinions. Sitting on my veranda that night, I tuned into the BBC World Service, the Voice of America and then listened to Radio Moscow; I gave the most credence to the BBC version of events, having been present when the events took place. Whether those refugees made it home I will never know.

Some time away

During a short break from Ibnat, I flew down to Addis Ababa to spend a few days having some time away. During the break, I was able to have a very special visit with renowned Australian gynaecologist, Dr Catherine Hamlin and her amazing staff at the Addis Ababa Fistula Hospital. Dr Hamlin had established the hospital in 1974, with her late Kiwi husband, Dr Reginald Hamlin. Ethiopian girls are often married off at a very young age, before they are fully developed, causing serious difficulties in childbirth. This causes obstetric fistulas (holes) between their bladders, vagina, and sometimes rectums, causing incontinence of both urine and faeces. Rejected by their husbands, these young women are doomed to live as social outcasts and in poverty for the rest of their lives. I was privileged to observe Dr Catherine and her team repair fistula damage and to hear the stories of some of these young girls. I will never forget the smiles on their faces when they received a new dress and were able to return to their home, not as outcasts but as beautiful women.

During my visit with Dr Catherine, I asked her if she would be willing to host Dr Ruth from Bannu Hospital, explaining that Ruth had been doing fistula operations in Bannu. Catherine agreed, I contacted Ruth, and everything fell into place; Ruth was able to spend time with Catherine at the Fistula hospital and on her return to Bannu, was able to put into practice the new fistula surgical skills she'd gained from Dr Catherine. The community of international medical aid workers wasn't large then, but the knowledge and skills they were able to share with one another through our network was amazing.

An unexpected proposal

While I was in Ethiopia, I received a most unexpected marriage proposal. I had met David (not his real name), an Englishman, in Bannu, where he used to volunteer on a regular basis at the hospital in Pakistan. Skilled in mechanics, welding and building, he was one of those practical people who could fix anything. David wanted to teach someone how to maintain the generator at Bannu Hospital and so, being a practical Kiwi girl, I volunteered. We spent many hours together in the generator shed as I learnt about its workings. Then, I went on assignment to Ethiopia and often wrote letters to my colleagues in Bannu, including David, signing off: 'Love, Barb,' as you do. Imagine my astonishment when I flew into Addis one day for a series of meetings and ran into David in the airport arrival gate. 'What are you doing here?' I asked. 'Barbara,' he said, 'I have come to help you in the camp, but I need to talk to you in private,' and so I suggested we speak in my hotel room. As I closed the door, he went down on one knee and said, 'Would you marry me? You obviously like me because you sign your letters 'Love, Barb.'' He added, 'Also, before you left Pakistan, you gave me a cup of coffee with the words; 'To Know You is to Love You' inscribed on the side. Flabbergasted, I told him I often signed my letters 'Love, Barb,' and the coffee cup came from the kitchen cupboard. 'I'm busy running a refugee camp hospital,' I told him. 'Marriage is the last thing on my mind.' David became upset and asked me to seriously consider his proposal and so I arranged to meet him in the hotel lobby after my meetings. That afternoon we had a long talk. I apologised if I'd sent him the wrong signals and gave him a firm, 'No.' A few days later I flew back to Ibnat Camp, and David spent a few weeks helping Aid Agencies in Addis before flying home. We parted as friends and were never to meet again.

33. As Kiwi as…

Ethiopia had been a challenging six-month interlude from my commitment to serving in Pakistan. Personally, I'd weathered yet another emotional storm with an unexpected marriage proposal. Professionally, I'd experienced at a deeper level the realities of disaster work in a country torn asunder by political tensions. A home visit was in order, and for that I had a travelling companion, Kipp, my Ibnat 'flatmate.' The pressure of this time was starting to show; in the middle of one of our last nights in Ibnat, Kipp had been woken up by me talking to myself. There I was on my bed perched on all fours, in an obviously distressed state. 'What are you doing, Barb?' she asked. 'Looking for starving children,' I replied, obviously not in a right state. Kipp assured me there were no starving children in our room and settled me down to sleep. Such was the strain of relief work.

Our contracts in Ethiopia had ended and we decided to return to New Zealand for a much-needed break, after which Kipp hoped to join me on the medical team at Bannu Hospital. Just before we left Ethiopia, the World Vision New Zealand Manager rang and asked, 'What are you most looking forward to when you get home?' Visions of smooth creamy ice-cream studded with crunchy golden-yellow sweets floated before our eyes, 'Hokey Pokey ice-cream!' we gleefully replied, thinking nothing more of it. Many hours later, the World Vision representative met us at Auckland airport with a plastic tub of Tip Top Hokey Pokey ice-cream and plastic spoons. It tasted even better than we'd imagined! Exhausted from our tediously long flight from Africa, we found news-hungry radio and TV crews waiting to interview us. We thanked the people of New Zealand and World Vision sponsors for their support and were delighted to be able to recount the heart-warming story of the lamb chops in a news item that was broadcast on national television that night. I was staying with my sister Wendy and her family in Auckland, and next morning I received a phone call from the managing director of Tip Top ice-cream; he'd seen the television interview and wanted to give us more hokey pokey ice-cream. He later filled my sister's freezer with ice-cream. My niece and nephew couldn't believe their luck! Kipp also received a generous share, which was delivered to her home in Whangarei.

After some rest, and a bit more ice cream, I checked in at the World Vision office in Auckland and did some more media interviews, before heading to my parents' home in Whakatane to spend time with family over Christmas, including nieces and nephews and their parents. I spent endless hours walking along the beautiful beach at Ohope, quietly reflecting on the situations I had left behind and adjusting to being home, although it would be only for a short time.

On the receiving end of care …

Refreshed after a two-month break in New Zealand, I returned to Bannu Hospital in January 1986. I was delighted that Kipp had joined our nursing team and was willing to pass her nursing skills on to Pakistani staff. Kipp made good use of her time there, and the hospital made good use of her skills in the coming months.

Purple Hands

We had arrived back during the cooler dry season but by July and August the weather in Bannu was brutally hot, with temperatures soaring to well over 35°C. Due to this extreme heat, the hospital was traditionally closed for the month of August and any patients who arrived were referred to the local government hospital. This meant that the staff were able to have a well-earned holiday. For us expats it meant getting out of Bannu and heading away to different parts of Pakistan for a break. That summer, Kipp, some friends and I decided to escape to Islamabad and stay a few nights with our British Embassy friends. However, during the early part of the trip, I wasn't feeling well, and my friends went on to another part of Pakistan without me.

After a few days of rest, I still felt unwell, and my embassy friends took me to a doctor. I was shocked and horrified to find that the blood test results showed possible typhoid; the doctor explained the best place for me to be would be in a hospital where they could watch me more closely. Soon afterwards, I was admitted to a private hospital with severe abdominal pain. Nurses inserted a saline drip into my arm and placed a 'Nil per mouth' notice above my head. There was some concern that I might have perforated my bowel (a serious complication of typhoid.) 'Call us when the drip needs changing,' the nurses said and left me to my own devices. I lay on the bed feeling ill and nauseated and so weak, I struggled to walk to the toilet. Fortunately, my embassy friends came in regularly during the day and assisted me to shower and make my bed and reassured me that this was the best medical facility available in Islamabad at that time. A doctor would call in every couple of days for a few minutes and I only saw the nurses when the drip needed changing, to give me pain relief and antibiotics. The days dragged on endlessly. After five days I was feeling slightly better and just wanted to get out of there. The pain was subsiding, the nausea was easing, and I was able to eat a small amount of soup which the embassy ladies brought in for me. The CMS UK insurance policy was covering the cost of my admission and I thought I would prefer to recover fully at one of the embassy houses rather than in this hospital. I managed to get a message to Kipp, who cut short her holiday to collect me and we went by taxi to our friend's embassy house.

Kipp had managed to buy a supply of Stemetil tablets and injections to combat nausea at one of the local shops in Islamabad and we decided the best way back to Bannu was to fly rather than travelling on the local buses. Arrangements were made for us to fly to Bannu via Peshawar the next day. At the airport, waves of nausea began to sweep over me, and we looked for somewhere for Kipp to inject me. The ladies' toilet seemed to be the only suitable place. Pulling down my baggy shalwar trousers, I leant over the toilet and Kipp injected Stemetil into my buttock while the toilet attendant gave us some strange looks. We boarded the plane to Peshawar for a two-hour flight and managed another Stemetil tablet before boarding another plane for the short flight to Bannu. In Bannu, the hospital car was there to meet us, and I was soon back in my bed, relieved to be lying down.

An hour or so after arriving home, I suddenly began to feel very strange. My jaw muscles were going into spasms, I couldn't open my mouth properly and my head and eyes were rolling uncontrollably upwards. Kipp, as a very experienced Kiwi nurse, immediately realised I was having an oculogyric crisis, a condition she had seen before in New Zealand. Dr Ruth wasn't in Bannu at the time, so Kipp spoke with the Pakistani doctor at the hospital, who suggested Valium, since the drug of choice for oculogyric crisis, Cogentin, was not available in the hospital. An ampoule of Valium was quickly given to Kipp and she immediately injected this into me. Thankfully, the crisis was averted, and I recovered well. Medical emergencies like mine are practically an everyday occurrence in developing countries, but sadly medical supplies are scant or non-existent for most people. Medics do the best they can with what they've got; but not every story has as happy an ending as mine.

Later, having been through this experience, I knew exactly what do while working in Somalia, when a colleague began to exhibit signs of an oculogyric crisis following a severe case of vomiting that had required Stemetil. Fortunately, we had a supply of Cogentin, which I gave her intravenously. She was relieved when her frightening symptoms subsided, as was I.

Unfortunately, this episode wasn't my only experience on the receiving end of care. Although the aid agencies and mission societies I worked with provided aid workers with medical insurance for any major emergencies, we often had to rely on local medical facilities to manage a situation, and the standard of health care and hygiene was invariably much lower than in New Zealand hospitals. We were fortunate to have experienced staff at our hospital in Bannu and I needed to call on their expertise one day when I developed a severe infection in my right index finger. Because the finger had become red, angry and extremely painful, the Pakistani hospital doctor injected a ring block anaesthetic into my finger, incised it and drained the pus to release the pressure. With a bandaged finger, I returned to work and over the next few days the wound improved. However, the infection returned with a vengeance some weeks later. The doctor put me on antibiotics and arranged to operate on my finger the following day to remove the deep-seated infection. This time I would have to have a general anaesthetic of chloroform and ether. This type of anaesthetic was no longer used in New Zealand and I was concerned about having it administered to me, but as the pain in my finger was so severe there wasn't really any other choice.

I lay on the operating table that day feeling petrified, wondering if I would be okay. A steel mask and a muslin cloth were placed on my face and the anaesthetic technician administered a light general anaesthetic via drops of chloroform, then drops of ether, with the combination being repeated until I was unconscious. The last thing I remember was smelling the chloroform and ether mixture and my head feeling like it was going to explode; I don't remember anything more. I woke sometime later to find myself in my own bed, with a few stitches in my finger and my hand swathed in a bandage. My finger soon recovered with the help of antibiotics, but colleagues later told me the technician had great difficulty ministering the anaesthetic and several nurses had to hold me down, as the anaesthetic took quite a while to work and I fought them until I was totally anaesthetized. Today, all I have to remind me of that experience is a small scar and a permanently numb area on my finger, as well as gratitude it hadn't been much worse.

You can take the Kiwi farm girl out of New Zealand…

Pennell Memorial Hospital was situated in the cantonment area just outside the city's solid mud-brick wall. On our days off, Kipp and I would venture into Bannu City and wander around the shops dressed in our salwar kameez, which we wore every day in Pakistan. Our trips were frowned upon by the Pakistani doctor, who feared we may be accosted or even kidnapped by men, but for me, making weekly visits to the bazaar was the only way I could stay sane. We never had any trouble from the thousands of men who flocked daily into Bannu City. I believe that this was because everyone knew that we were part of the Pennell Memorial Hospital staff. Our trips into the city were often on the premise of choosing new fabrics to bring to the local tailor, who would make us shalwar kameez and dupattas for the many Pakistani weddings we were invited to. On these occasions, we'd choose much fancier fabric than for our work salwar kameez, and one of the many female Pakistani hospital staff who lived nearby would always guide us on the latest fashion for weddings. These special occasions and trips outside of the hospital compound helped to make life balanced, bearable and a bit more fun.

Eventually, needing to do something to break up our day to day routine, I decided to bring a bit of Kiwi culture into our lives at the hospital. As a child, I had been very keen on raising pet lambs, and after some discussion with Kipp, I suggested to my colleagues that we have some sheep in the large back yard of our house, who could help keep the grass down, and would also be a source of meat; after much discussion it was finally agreed that I would buy one pregnant ewe. So, one Friday morning, Kipp and I set off for the sheep market at the Bannu bazaar, accompanied by a male staff member. This was strictly a male area, and we were clearly the focus of attention. We wandered around, checking out the sheep and examining them carefully, and to the shock and amusement of the hundreds of men, I bought one female sheep. We flagged down a horse-driven cart (tonga) which was the main form of transport in Bannu for those who didn't own a car, tied up the sheep's legs, laid her across our laps, and headed off home. We named the sheep Woofie and she settled in well. We'd been assured she was pregnant and so we waited and waited. Sure enough, a few months later we came home to find a lamb at her side, which we would name Spurlai, meaning 'spring' in Pashtu. This was the beginning of our sheep legacy.

When the time was right, we mated Spurlai with a ram owned by the wife of a staff member, and in due course another lamb was born. Our flock grew to two sheep and two lambs. But then another issue arose. How would we shear our sheep? Surgical scissors did the trick, and Kipp and I sheared our small flock on our day off. We sold the wool and donated the proceeds towards a new midwifery unit at the hospital. The sheep saga continued. One day, I discovered that one of our ewes had given birth to a lamb but failed to deliver the placenta. As a midwife, I had removed retained placentas in human patients, and so I decided to remove the ewe's placenta. Handling a frightened ewe in my small bathroom wasn't easy, and she complained noisily. I had my hand inside the ewe and was feeling for the placenta, when I looked up, feeling someone watching. Dr Ruth was looking at me with a stunned expression on her face. 'I'm doing a manual placenta removal,' I explained. Dr Ruth shook her head in disbelief and left. Both the ewe and I were relieved when I delivered the placenta.

No sooner had I finished than there was a knock on the bathroom door: 'Sister Barbara, come!' It was the night guard calling me to a delivery case at the hospital. I hastily tied up the ewe, washed my arms and hands, changed my bloodied salwar kameez for my salwar kameez uniform and headed over to the hospital to deliver a healthy baby boy and placenta. Returning hours later, I cleaned up the bloodied bathroom, which looked like a war zone. I headed for bed, reminding myself that next morning I had two patients to check; a mother and a sheep (and both of their babies). Both recovered well.

On another occasion a birthing ewe developed a prolapse. This was partially hanging out and attracting flies, which caused infection. I tried attaching a sanitary pad to hold her prolapse in, but to no avail. So, I decided to approach Dr Ruth, a skilled surgeon who had performed many operations on women with vaginal, rectal and uterine prolapses. 'Dr Ruth, what are you doing on your day off?' I asked. 'Why?' she responded. 'You know Bibi the lovely tribal woman with the prolapse you operated on a few days ago? She's doing so well…and I'm wondering if you could do a similar operation on my ewe? She has a prolapse which I am not able to keep clean and without an operation she'll have to be put down.' Dr Ruth was speechless. 'I'm happy to pay for the suture material, local anaesthetic and ring pessary,' I continued. 'I'll think about it and let you know,' Dr Ruth replied. Later she came to me and said, 'I will try.' Then history was made that day on the back steps outside the kitchen door when she repaired my ewe's prolapse. Both the sheep and Bibi recovered well with Dr Ruth's expert care. Dr Ruth and a colleague later wrote an article about our kitchen-door surgery event which was published in the *British Medical Journal*. People from all over the world responded, saying how much they enjoyed the article.

Time for self-care

Caring for my sheep was one thing; caring for myself was becoming harder. I was beginning to dread my monthly periods as each month the pain was getting worse. I was taking ever-increasing pain relief so I could keep on working. Because I didn't want to bother anyone at the hospital, I bought pain tablets over the counter at the local bazaar. I knew that taking so many pills would affect my kidneys in the long term but brushed the matter aside. My periods were becoming more frequent and intense. The pain was getting so severe that I finally decided to do something about it. I talked with Dr Ruth, who listened with concern and planned for me to see a male gynaecologist in Peshawar, our nearest major city. The gynaecologist asked me lots of questions and after examining me, suggested it would be helpful if he carried out a laparoscopy to find out what was going on. Scans were not heard of at this time, and especially not in Pakistan. I agreed to the laparoscopy.

At the appointed time, I arrived at the private hospital for the procedure. I was shown into the maternity ward and told to sit and wait. I became very concerned, as I expected to be treated in a private consulting room, not a maternity ward with labouring women. I felt very uncomfortable sitting in the ward with the women, two to a bed. A nurse arrived and told me to roll up my sleeve, which I did very hesitantly. I was even more anxious when she went over to a trolley and lifted the lid off a container of needles and syringes which were floating in some liquid. She assembled the syringe, attached the needle, and proceeded to draw up whatever was about to be injected into my arm. I asked her what this was for, and not understanding her reply in Urdu, I was beginning to become very agitated. The specialist doctor arrived and informed me that I would soon be walking down to the theatre. He also asked if I would mind if some student doctors were present during the procedure. 'Okay,' I said, and began walking down the corridor heading to the theatre. A colleague was with me and as I walked into the theatre in my street clothes, and in bare feet having already removed my shoes, I turned to my colleague and said, 'Please pray, and if I am not out in thirty minutes, come in and get me.' As I looked around the theatre, I couldn't help noticing the dust on the anaesthetic trolley. I climbed up on to the bed. The surgeon arrived, prepared my skin and injected local anaesthetic into the area below my belly button. I remember terrible pain, then …. nothing. When I woke up, I was lying on a stretcher in the consultant's office. The consultant was standing over me. 'How are you feeling?' he asked. 'Very sore' I replied. 'Barbara, you were the most difficult patient I've ever had. I perform this operation regularly and I gave you the same amount of local anaesthetic as I give the Pakistani ladies when I do tubal ligations or laparoscopy surgery on them. 'But you kicked and screamed and tried to get off the table; we had to knock you right out.' I looked at him and I remember saying, 'You get up on the table and I will give you some local and then put a knife into your stomach and we will see what you do.'

He went on to say, 'I have found endometriosis, and would suggest that you look at having a laparotomy to see how extensive it is. I can do such an operation here or you could go to England. I suggest you talk with Dr Ruth. I will send you a full report.'

I thanked him, climbed down off the trolley and left. Once we got back to the hotel where we were staying, I decided to have a look at my wound. I lifted my top and was surprised to see a plaster with a Mickey Mouse face on it across the incision. I gently lifted it off and was shocked to see the suture was thick nylon reminiscent of my New Zealand fishing line. When the report on my condition arrived, I discussed it with Dr Ruth and decided I should head to the United Kingdom for further investigations. As New Zealand and British hospitals had a reciprocal medical care arrangement, I was assured that it would all be fine.

I flew down to Islamabad and British Embassy friends arranged for me to fly to the UK for possible surgery. One of the embassy staff was flying there at the same time and so she travelled with me, which was reassuring. CMS UK, the British mission society I worked for, had arranged an appointment for me at the Chelsea Women's Hospital in London. On arrival at Heathrow, I duly filled in the arrival card, giving surgery as my reason for coming to England. At the immigration counter I was asked the reason for my visit. 'For surgery,' I said. 'It has all been arranged at Chelsea Women's hospital in London.' I explained that I would be staying with a friend in London, and that her address was on my card. 'Where do you live?' the immigration officer asked. 'Pakistan,' I replied. 'We don't have any reciprocal arrangement with Pakistan,' he said sternly. I tried to explain that I was working in Pakistan, but my home was New Zealand, but to no avail. 'Go to one side and wait,' he ordered. An officious-looking woman arrived. 'Come with me!' she instructed. Accompanied by my Embassy friend, I followed her down long corridors and was told to go into a small room and wait. Puzzled and confused, I asked them to tell my friend waiting to meet me in the arrivals hall that I was being detained. They said they would. Feeling like an illegal immigrant, I sat in the small room with my travelling companion. It felt cold and impersonal. People walked up and down the corridor. 'What if they send me back to Pakistan?' I wondered.

By this time, I was feeling a lot of abdominal pain and so I asked for a glass of water and took a couple of Severdol tablets from my bazaar supply. I couldn't understand why I was being subjected to this distressing situation. Finally, my embassy friend had to go as she was catching another flight. 'I'll be fine,' I said, unconvincingly. 'Thanks for your support and we'll catch up again in Pakistan.' I had no idea what was going to happen next. The woman official asked me why I was in England, and I explained the situation again. 'You'll have to see our doctor,' she said. 'Fine,' I replied. 'I'm happy to see a doctor.' After waiting for an interminable amount of time, I was called in to see the doctor, where I explained what was wrong, why I was here and that I had an appointment with a doctor. He asked me the doctor's name and when I said, 'Dr Wright, (not her real name) the Mission Society's doctor,' everything suddenly changed. 'Oh, I was at medical school with her,' said the doctor, our paths still cross occasionally. I'm sure she'll have everything under control. You are free to go.'

He called the immigration lady in from outside. 'Go with her and she will get your passport stamped,' he said. 'I hope things go well.' I thanked him and then went back to immigration, got my passport stamped and was shown out into a small room where my friend Wendy was waiting. Boy, was I pleased to see her!

The next day I attended my appointment at the hospital and the surgery, a laparotomy, was booked for two days' time. Finally, after many years of pain, the diagnosis of severe endometriosis was made. Treatment was started, and after a recovery time I returned to Pakistan. The surgeon told me he would be happy to see me when I was back in the UK and suggested I stay in touch. I continued with the medication which helped a little to manage my condition.

A death in the family

Personal medical problems pale into insignificance in the face of family suffering. At such times, distance becomes a huge issue, a painful separation from those you love most. Communication with New Zealand was a complicated matter at the best of times in the days long before cell phones, satellite phones or faxes. If we wanted to make a phone call to New Zealand, we had to go to the exchange centre in Bannu and get the staff there to make a call. It often took most of the morning, so we didn't do this very often. The main form of communication was via hand-written aerogrammes and these could take weeks to reach their destination. Then there were the telegrams, a more direct, urgent form of communication. These usually brought bad news, and we dreaded receiving them.

I received a telegram when I was working in Bannu. That afternoon, I was heading over to the hospital to begin my shift when an elderly postman cycled up to the gate and spoke with the gardener. He handed over an envelope saying, 'Sister Barbara.' The gardener came and gave me the envelope. I opened it, dreading what I was about to read. There it was, the bad news. My grandmother Mabel, my mother's mother, had died. She had moved to Whakatane to be near my parents after her husband, my grandfather, had died some years earlier. The finality of the news overwhelmed me. I knew my family would be gathering and planning her funeral. It was times like that when I felt so far away and so alone. With my emotions in a turmoil, I put the envelope into my pocket and as I walked across to the hospital, as I was about to go on duty, I reminisced about my grandmother who had been supportive of my nursing and my overseas work. I spent the afternoon busy in the hospital, delivering babies and working alongside the staff, and then headed back to the bungalow for dinner. Kipp noticed that I was a bit quieter than usual and asked if I was okay. I said I was fine. After dinner I went into my room, struggling a bit, but also not wanting to share how I was really feeling. Kipp followed me in, and asked again, concerned for my well-being. I said nothing and handed her the envelope with the telegram. She read it and then gave me a big hug. We spent time together in prayer. Later, I felt able to tell the others what had happened. They were very supportive. My family wrote and told me all about my grandmother's funeral. It brought tears to my eyes. How sad I was not to have been there. Both grandmothers had died while I was working overseas.

Goodbye, Bannu!

My time in Bannu was coming to an end. I had learnt a lot, gained a huge amount of experience, and met some truly amazing people who had so generously welcomed me, the first Kiwi girl to work in Bannu, putting up with me and my different ways. During my time there I had been involved in helping to set up an under-fives vaccination clinic to try to reduce the number of killer childhood diseases; I had helped in training a number of Pakistani staff in midwifery; and had worked hard with my colleagues in the planning and building of a new midwifery unit. I had really enjoyed my time in Bannu. After five and a half years it was time to move on. I realized that I needed a change, as did the expat team I had been working with. I was sad to be leaving, but for me it was the right time. I had received a letter from a colleague I had worked with in Somalia, telling me that there was a position for a matron in a remote hospital in northern Kenya; this would be the next chapter in God's plan for my life.

34. Back Under African Skies: Kenya, 1988

I was back in Africa, working for a Finnish mission, when I suddenly found myself in the midst of my worst nightmare: I had just completed my first two weeks of Kiswahili language instruction in Nairobi, and was behind the wheel of a mission car, returning to our Finnish team houses in Nakuru. Driving in Kenya is challenging at the best of times, so I was driving cautiously, at a safe speed. A language teacher had asked for a ride to a certain town, I had just dropped him off, and was continuing my journey. It was mid-afternoon, and I was driving on my own in unfamiliar surroundings and navigating tarmac roads full of large potholes through villages with throngs of people who had a complete lack of concern for oncoming traffic. As I drove, the advice of seasoned missionaries was uppermost in my mind; the rules around traffic accidents were very clear: 'If you have an accident and hit someone when driving, don't stop. Drive straight to the nearest police station and report the accident.' My missionary colleagues, many of whom had been in Kenya for years, insisted it was too risky for a white person to stop and inquire if someone was injured, as the gathering crowd could turn on the driver. I had stored this information away, hoping I'd never be in such a situation.

As I approached a small village, I noticed passengers getting on a bus on the left-hand side of the road. Seeing a man and an elderly woman standing on the right-hand side of the road, I slowed down. Suddenly I saw a flash of colour and heard a thump. Looking in the rear vision mirror, I saw something flying. It looked like a human form. The words of those missionaries resounded in my ears: 'If you have an accident, don't stop! Go to the nearest police station,' and so I kept driving for another hundred yards. But something made me stop and turn back. Terrified, I cried out to God for protection. With my heart pounding, I arrived at the spot. The elderly woman I'd noticed a few minutes ago was on the ground. Kneeling to examine her, I saw that she was bleeding profusely from a major head injury and a badly damaged ankle. A man who was leaning over her, in clear English said 'This is my mother. Can you help us?' he pleaded. 'We were crossing the road to catch the bus and she walked straight into the path of your car, I told her to wait but she didn't. Please help us!' he begged. 'The nearest hospital is in Nakuru.' I hesitated. I had already broken the rules. But as a human being, as a Christian aid worker, I decided to listen to my heart. To this day, I believe I made the right decision.

Her son and I lifted the woman onto the back seat of my vehicle, and I instructed him to hold her head up to assist her breathing, while keeping pressure on his mother's head wound to help stem the bleeding. Shaking like a leaf, I got into the driver's seat and drove off. Over the next few anxious, prayerful hours, I was constantly glancing in the rear vision mirror, asking how she was doing, while trying to keep calm and focus on the road. When we finally arrived at Nakuru Hospital, I parked the car and, covered in blood, ran down the corridor asking for help. The staff was busy and every one of them ignored me. Sobbing, I stood in the corridor feeling increasingly desperate. I'd hit a woman and she had very serious head and ankle injuries. Thoughts tormented me 'Why didn't you just keep driving? You may regret your decision to stop and help!' Then God sent an angel in the form of a Kenyan hospital cleaner. Listening to my predicament, she offered to get a trolley. We fetched the trolley and trundled it down the seemingly endless corridor and out to the car where the patient's son was waiting anxiously. A crowd had gathered, talking amongst themselves and staring at me. As the only white person and the apparent perpetrator of the crime, I felt very vulnerable. We lifted the woman onto the trolley, wheeled her down the corridor to the emergency room and I gave the staff a brief account of what had happened. Then I explained to the son I was going to my team house near the hospital to get a colleague who would help. 'Thank you,' said the son, taking my hand. 'You've saved my mother's life.' With tears streaming down our faces, we stood in the emergency room and I prayed for his mother and for both of us.

Fortunately, two senior missionaries were at the team house when I arrived there, and between sobs, I explained what had happened. They were quick to reassure me and said, 'We need to go to the police station and report the accident.' I quickly showered and changed out of my bloodstained clothes and one of them drove me to the police station. However, the policeman said I needed to go to the police station nearest to where the accident happened. So, my colleague and I drove back to the hospital to collect the woman's son. We then drove for some hours to the police station nearest to the scene of the accident.

Both the patient's son and I were asked to fill out papers stating what had happened. The policeman told me to add to what I had written that I'd been driving fast and dangerously in my statement. 'But that's not the truth!' I retorted. Thankfully the son supported me. 'My mother ran out in front of the car. It was my mother's fault,' he asserted. But his words fell on deaf ears. Flicking through the pages of my passport, the policeman said coldly, 'Either you write that you were driving fast and dangerously, or I will arrest you and place you in a police cell. I can assure you; you will come out of the cell very different from how you went in.'

Fear overwhelmed me; despite all the warnings I'd been given, I had landed myself in deep trouble. In desperation, I cried out and asked God to help me. For the second time that day, an angel appeared. He came in the guise of a senior police officer who entered the room and asked me who I was and what had happened. I explained I was the new matron of the Kapedo mission hospital north of Nakuru and had been in Nairobi learning Kiswahili and was driving back to Nakuru when the accident occurred. He listened carefully and said, 'Barbara, I know the hospital well and the staff. Don't worry – go home now. Bring your car to the police station tomorrow and we will examine it. Thank you for helping this lady and her son.'

My fear evaporated. I felt enormously grateful that God had heard my prayer for help. We returned to Nakuru, somewhat reassured, although I wasn't out of the woods yet. The next morning, my colleague and I took my car to the police station and found that there was no damage at all. I notified my mission leaders, who were based in Nairobi, of the accident and was driven back to Nairobi the next day to complete the paperwork and be interviewed by a private investigator who then took over the case. I rang friends in New Zealand and the United Kingdom and asked them to pray. No charges were laid against me.

I was advised not to visit the mother in hospital, and took the advice this time, but staff assured me she was making good progress. Months later, the son approached me at a church service in Nakuru and gave me a big hug, saying, 'My mother is recovering. Thank you for saving her life. Without your help she would have died.'

That horrific baptism by fire resulted in many direct conversations between God and me, with me asking, 'Why me?' I thought about what my life would be if I hadn't dropped that teacher off en route back to Nakuru; the accident wouldn't have happened. I was really struggling and prayed daily that God would give me His peace, which He did, eventually. In hindsight now, I wouldn't change anything, but initially I struggled to get into a car, and I refused to drive.

Some weeks later, while back in Nairobi continuing my language lessons, God sent across my path a Christian woman from America who was staying in the same hostel as me in Nairobi. One morning at breakfast she said, 'I was praying early this morning and God laid you on my heart and asked if I was willing to be an instrument of healing in your life. He also showed me that you have recently been through a very traumatic situation.' 'You are amazing, God!' I thought, as I told her about the accident. As she prayed for me, God reached into my life and removed the trauma. Because of the healing I gained through this, not only was I able to get behind the wheel again, but I was able to continue to fulfil God's call to be a Christian aid worker in the developing world.

Kapedo Mission Hospital

Aside from this distressing situation, it was good to be back in Africa, although my route to get there was a little roundabout. Most aid workers quickly become members of the 'disaster crisis network,' and we all got our news through the grapevine, which back then was via letters from friends and mission groups (nowadays it would be via social media). One day, while I was working in Bannu, I had received a letter from a Finnish doctor I had worked with in Somalia, Dr Sven, not his real name telling me that a Finnish mission he was working for needed an experienced nurse-midwife to be matron. Dr Sven was the only doctor working in this Kapedo Mission Hospital, in a small village a few hours north of Nakuru in Kenya. He was struggling with the workload and was looking for someone with extensive experience to assist him. (Sven's wife and his mother also lived in Kapedo, but they weren't involved in the medical work.) So, after negotiating a contract with the Finnish mission and completing the paperwork, I headed to Kenya. An African proverb says: If you ever sleep under an African sky, you will always return to Africa. I was looking forward to fulfilling this in my new role.

Dr Sven and his wife met me at Nairobi Airport, and we headed for the team house in Nakuru, a bustling city three hours from Nairobi full of Indian shopkeepers, Somalians, and Kenyans. Our three-bedroom house in Nakuru had a bathroom with a bath and a large Finnish sauna in the garden (Unlike the Finns, I preferred the bath to the sauna.). This house later became my haven, a welcoming place to stay when we came to Nakuru for a break from the isolation of Kapedo. But Kapedo was to be my home for the next two years. To get there, we drove for four or five hours, first on a tarmac road and then on desert tracks and through small riverbeds, dry at that time of year, but raging torrents in the rainy season.

En route, we often passed groups of three or four small boys, miles from aywhere, usually with a stick, a few goats, a couple of cows and some very scrawny sheep. It was their job to make sure that their animals found bushes to eat, and that wild dogs didn't get them before they returned them to their parents' homes in the late afternoons. The boys were a welcome distraction during the long, hot, and dusty trip to Kapedo, which left us all tired, hot and dusty ourselves by the time we arrived. The village consisted of a couple of shops, a post office of sorts and three well-constructed western-looking houses where the missionaries lived, close to the concrete block building which could loosely be called a 'hospital.' As I took this all in, I reflected that once again I was in a new place, in the middle of nowhere, at a disadvantage with my language skills – no knowledge of Finnish and very limited Kiswahili – and that this was certainly going to be an interesting assignment. I could only put one foot in front of the other and see where this new journey would take me.

I was shown to my house, a building made of concrete with a veranda at the front. This veranda was to become one of my favourite places, especially when temperatures rose, making it too hot to stay inside. My house made up of two bedrooms, a lounge and a basic bathroom, was situated on a hill overlooking a deep valley through which a small river flowed, and fed a large, hot waterfall. As I came in, the house girl gave me a warm welcome, but communication was going to be a challenge. She had very little English and I had very little Kiswahili. Next to my house was my own in ground swimming pool. Between my swimming pool and the doctor's house was a shed, and inside the shed was – you've guessed right – another sauna! (After all, it was a Finnish ministry.) I spent many late afternoons and early evenings floating in my private swimming pool, looking over the valley below (but didn't use the sauna, as it was something which I didn't really enjoy).

The telephone exchange was just across the road from my house and the lady in charge assured me in broken English that she could connect me to anyone anywhere in the world. The telephone system consisted of a mass of wires and numerous car batteries, neatly lined up on the ground, 'Yeah, right!' I thought. A few weeks later I had the chance to check this, when I decided to ring my parents, who were living in Edgecumbe, a small town in New Zealand's North Island. I gave the operator the number and she connected a few wires. I wasn't feeling confident. But we got a dial tone! She keyed in the phone number, and a few minutes later I was talking to my parents. Amazing! The lady wasn't sure what to charge me, but I paid what I thought was a reasonable amount.

Despite the isolation of Kapedo, and the difficulty of getting building supplies, the early Finnish missionaries, many of whom had engineering skills, certainly used their skills as they constructed the hospital and staff accommodation on a ridge above a river which was part of the geothermal area running through that part of Kenya, from Lake Turkana in the north down to a thermal area close to Lake Nakuru.

To get to the waterfall, I had to climb down a track and then walk through the river, which was knee deep for most of the year. The area where the water from the waterfall flowed into the river was hot, while the rest of the river was cool. There were many crocodiles who lounged in the sun on the banks of the river and every now and then they would slide themselves into the cooler water, which meant that the local people, who bathed in the cooler water, had to be very careful. The expats preferred the heated area of the water, so we had no concerns about the crocodiles. Because the locals didn't like the crocodiles or the hot waterfall, and the crocodiles didn't like the hot water, it became a favourite spot of the expats.

Nature had provided me with my own natural massage apparatus; the force of that hot waterfall was so strong I could only bear to stand under it for a few minutes. But the pounding on my neck and back was a great form of massage, especially after a busy day in the hospital, or after a three-day medical safari. I frequently wandered down to the waterfall with my toilet bag to wash my hair and enjoy an intensive massage before lying in the warm pools to the side or sitting in the hot pools that surrounded the waterfall. Kapedo had its charms.

The Kenyan Nursing Council and me

Before arriving in Kenya, I had applied to the Kenyan Nursing Council to become registered as a nurse and midwife in that country. Some weeks later I was asked to come to Nairobi for an interview. At the appointed time, I turned up at the Nursing Council office and waited to be called into the chief nurse's office. Walking into the room, I noticed there were no chairs, so I stood in front of the three unsmiling Kenyans who were seated behind a huge table. 'Hopefully this won't last too long,' I thought. They began to fire questions at me. 'Why was I in Kenya?' 'Where had I come from?' They asked extensively about my training in New Zealand and my nursing experience. Although I had sent them this information prior to the interview, I politely answered their questions. It was tiring, as I was not offered a chair to sit down on and after two hours of questions, I began to wonder just what I would be asked next. Finally, they said, 'You are not qualified to work as a nurse here in Kenya. Your training isn't up to Kenyan standards. If you want to work here, you will have to do more training in our hospitals, and in our delivery service, as well as our public health programme.'

I couldn't believe my ears: I was a New Zealand-registered nurse midwife, a registered nurse in Tasmania and a registered nurse in the United Kingdom. Those countries had accepted my training, but Kenya would not. I must have looked stunned, as one of the interview panel members said to me, 'If a Kenyan nurse came to your country, they would have to do more training before they would be registered. You white people think you can come and work here and walk straight in.' What she said was probably true, but despite that, I wasn't prepared to do any more training. I simply wanted to get on with the job I'd been appointed to. They told me to go away and think about it and get back to them.

Feeling overwhelmed, I left the room and walked down the stairs. Dr Sven was waiting for me. He was shocked but not surprised when I told him what had happened. We headed back to the guest house where we were staying and talked more over supper. Three American nurses staying at the guest house were in the same situation I was in; two had decided to go home. The third had agreed to undertake more training in Kenya and had some interesting stories to tell of her experiences working in one of the hospitals in Nairobi, which confirmed what I imagined training here might be like; of oxygen masks in the intensive care unit being in such short supply that the patients shared masks, of a shortage of sterile water resulting in tap water being used in its place, and more. The stories were enlightening, to say the least. 'There must be another way I can work in Kenya,' I thought.

The next day, on our way back to Nakuru, Dr Sven and I called into the office of the Provincial Medical Officer of Health (PMO), who Dr Sven knew well. He invited us both into his office, where Dr Sven explained the situation, mentioning the huge difficulties the Kapedo hospital faced, not only in getting expatriate nurses, but also in getting Kenyan nurses; Kapedo was so isolated, people didn't want to work there. The PMO then asked me to share my training and work history, which I did, slightly more comfortably than I had the day before. After some thought he said, 'I am happy for you to work in Kapedo and am pleased you have come. You can work under my authority and everything will be okay.' We thanked him and left his office. Once again, the connections Dr Sven had made had helped me through a very difficult situation.

Dr Sven wasn't exaggerating when he had described the limits of the hospital in Kapedo, which was very small and very basic. It was staffed by three local Kenyan nurses, a handful of assistants, Dr Sven, and me. It consisted of three rooms where we looked after patients, and a small theatre (where I delivered babies and Dr Sven performed minor surgery, including occasional eye procedures) none of which had glass in the windows. Our supply of medications was limited, the power supply was a hit and miss affair, and the hot water was occasional. However, the hospital was needed, and appreciated, by the locals in such an isolated location.

Two communities used the hospital: the Turkanas and the Pokot. These nomadic tribes wandered the desert looking after their cows, sheep and goats, with poison-tip bows and arrows as their main form of protection from wild animals or their enemies. Members of both tribes often presented at the hospital with malaria, snake bite, diarrhoea and vomiting, pneumonia, cuts, broken limbs, and skin and eye diseases. At times, there was tension between these two tribes and violence erupted, but we remained neutral at the hospital, of course, and treated all who came to us for help. Being an experienced midwife, especially given my comprehensive training in Pakistan, I was often called to the hospital at night to assist with complex deliveries. Traditional birth attendants delivered most of the babies in the local area, and mothers only came to the hospital when they were having difficulties. At such times, I was escorted to the hospital by the night guard (a Turkana man, wearing a bow and arrows and only a bit of leather to cover his private parts). On such calls, I performed a number of forceps deliveries which saved patients the four to five-hour drive to Nakuru hospital, on a road so bad in parts that it had to be driven on tracks, crossing numerous riverbeds; an extremely difficult drive during the wet season. We were thankful we were able to be there for these patients who would have no other options.

One day, I was on duty when a woman delivered a stillborn baby. When a person died, they were buried in an area some distance from the hospital. In this case, family members declined to come to the cemetery, but I offered to drive the guard, a nurse and the dead baby there. Off we went, with Kenyan Nurse George carrying the baby, carefully wrapped in a piece of cloth. When we arrived in the designated area, driving became more difficult. There were no signposts we could see indicating where the graves were, or even that we were in a cemetery. Guided by Nurse George, I cautiously drove around, looking for a suitable place to bury the baby. Suddenly the front wheel on the passenger side sank into a deep hole and the vehicle stalled. Nurse George had a very worried look on his face. We both managed to climb out of the vehicle, but George refused to investigate the hole our vehicle had fallen into. Slowly and apprehensively, I made my way to the passenger's side and looked in. My suspicions were confirmed: the hole was a grave. The front tyre was probably a good two to three feet down in the grave. I hesitantly investigated the hole, expecting to see a body or even a skeleton. To my relief, I saw nothing but dirt. 'It's okay,' I said to him. 'There's no body.' Warily, George approached the hole and plucked up the courage to look inside. Nothing. 'What do we do now?' I asked. 'We should bury the baby. Then we'll need to get the vehicle out of the grave,' he replied. 'How?' I wondered aloud. It would need a crane or some very big trucks. George dug a grave; I said a prayer as we buried the baby. Then we returned to our problem. There were no other vehicles at the mission hospital and all the expatriates were out or staying at the team houses in Nakuru. If I'd been in New Zealand, I could have rung the AA (Automobile Association)! Even if I'd rung a garage in Nakuru a good four to five hours away, I don't think anyone would have come. We sat there, stranded. Suddenly, Nurse

George had an idea: There was an army base not far away. 'They'll have some vehicles and maybe they could help us.'

We locked our 4-wheel-drive vehicle and started walking to the camp which was some kilometres away. With my limited Swahili, I was reassured to have Nurse George with me, and when we arrived at the camp, being the only white person around, I was openly stared at. Nurse George explained who I was and what our problem was. 'The front passenger side wheel of our hospital vehicle has fallen into a grave. We are not able to get the vehicle out. Would you be able to come and tow us?' The soldiers exchanged glances, partly amused and partly apprehensive at the talk of graves. Nurse George explained we had examined the grave and couldn't see any bodies, which brought some relief to the soldiers. After more conversing and more glances at me, some soldiers agreed to see what they could do to help. We set off riding in an army truck, followed by two others, carrying more soldiers. When we arrived at the cemetery, two of the braver soldiers walked towards the vehicle and cautiously peered into the hole. More discussion ensued before a large wire rope attached to the winch on the army truck was tied to the tow-bar on the back of our Land Rover, and we all stood clear as the winch, which was attached to a small engine, was switched on. There was sudden eruption of smoke and an ear-splitting noise. I covered my ears and held my breath as slowly, oh so slowly, the winch dragged our vehicle out of the hole. Fortunately, there was no damage to the vehicle; just some damage to my pride. We could breathe easily again. With smiles all around, handshakes and many *asanta sana* (thank you), I jumped into the driver's seat and we drove back to the hospital, another adventure under our belts, another disaster avoided.

We often had to do our work off site, and in challenging locations. After some weeks in Kapedo, I felt confident enough to accompany a couple of Kenyan nurses and a driver on their regular medical safaris. We would load up the 4-wheel-drive with medical supplies, food and water, a spare tyre, diesel, a blanket and pillow and head into remoter areas for three or four days. The rough roads – often more like goat tracks – went for miles into the barren, isolated regions. The dust in the dry season and the mud and raging rivers in the wet season provided challenges enough for a lifetime. There were no garages, no breakdown services, and we had a basic radio which didn't work most of the time. Once we left Kapedo, we were on our own in the vast outdoors. Before heading out, we would spend time in prayer, asking God for His protection. We never knew what we would encounter, whether medical emergencies, problems with vehicles, or issues with our own health.

On one such medical safari, we travelled for several hours towards a remote Pokot village. These nomadic people and their animals traditionally wandered in search of food and water, but at times, some members stayed in areas near rivers where there were grass and shrubs for their stock to eat. Occasionally, if the land was suitable, these groups would grow maize and beans for the tribe. On our arrival in one of these temporary villages, we were greeted by village leaders and told there was a medical emergency. Nurse George listened and explained to me that there was a woman in labour who was experiencing difficulties. Nurse George suggested I examine the woman and confirm what was needed while he stood outside the makeshift shelter and explained to the Pokot traditional birth attendant that I was experienced and wanting to help. After being given the visual 'once-over,' I was ushered inside, along with Nurse George as translator, who stayed out of sight of the women. After some discussion, the woman in advanced labour agreed to let me examine her. The foetal heartbeat was audible and regular, and the mother was 6cm dilated, but the green meconium discharge I could see indicated the baby was in trouble. I asked Nurse George to explain that we needed to get the woman to the nearest local hospital two hours away by vehicle but more than a day's walk on foot. After more discussion, mostly between the men, rather than with the labouring woman or the traditional birth attendant, the decision was taken to transport her to this medical facility. We loaded the patient, her husband and the traditional birth attendant onto the vehicle. With the guys sitting in the front of the vehicle, and the women jammed in the back, we set off.

We were under pressure to get the patient to the hospital as fast as we could. Frustratingly, the condition of the goat track of a road severely limited our speed. The bouncing around perhaps was helping to progress the woman's contractions which were getting much stronger, but there was also an alarming increase in the amount of meconium flowing. I knew we were in trouble. I had to take matters in hand. Asking the driver to stop, I told men to get out of the vehicle, as I needed to examine the woman. Nurse George explained to the patient, and after listening for the foetal heartbeat, now very faint, I examined her and found her fully dilated. So, with the next contraction we all encouraged her to push. She gave it her best but, with four more contractions and more meconium, and still no baby, I had no choice. I asked Nurse George to fetch the forceps from my maternity bag. I drew up some local anaesthetic and injected it around the area to be cut. Just before the next contraction, I applied the forceps. As the contraction began, I performed a large episiotomy. As the contraction built up, I began to pull on the forceps and pray. After a huge effort on the patient's part, together with a huge effort on mine, I managed to get the baby's head out. Removing the forceps and checking for the cord, I delivered the baby. Sadly, the new-born baby was very floppy. I grabbed the stethoscope and listened. There was no heartbeat. I kept my stethoscope on the baby's chest for some time; the baby was not breathing. I looked at Nurse George wordlessly. They could see from my face and my actions, that the baby had died. Tears welled up in the patient's eyes. I cut the cord, wrapped the baby and handed it to the mother. I could feel her pain. For some time, nothing was said. I delivered the placenta and stitched up the episiotomy.

Then I stood up and asked Nurse George to translate as I offered my love and support to the mother. I felt extremely sad, wondering as I always did if I could have done anything different. If I had been in a modern hospital in the west, maybe the answer would have been 'yes.' The medical services out here in the back of beyond were poles apart from there, and I'd made my decisions according to the resources available to me. Although I had done my best, it was very hard to accept that a baby was dead. I signalled to Nurse George and we both walked some distance away. I asked him, 'What should we do now?' 'I will ask the husband,' he said. The husband asked that we dispose of the baby over the bank. He said there was no point in taking it home. Mortified, I said to Nurse George, 'We can't!' I imagined the headline in the national daily paper: Western aid worker nurse throws dead Pokot baby over the bank. The Kenyan Nurses' Council wouldn't be happy either! I talked to Nurse George and finally said, 'Let's take the parents and baby back to their village and they can take care of the baby as they prefer.' We arrived back in the village and were greeted by the villagers. Once the patient was settled back in her shelter, Nurse George spoke to the elders, we said our good-byes and left. I had mixed emotions as we drove away, but I knew that I had done my best.

Barbara Walker

On the Sudanese border

As part of our traveling medical service, I also accompanied Dr Sven, a skilled eye surgeon, on several eye safaris. We would load up the Land Rover with supplies and surgical equipment and travel to remote areas where he would carry out eye surgery, including cataract procedures. I continued to do occasional trachoma operations, often with the patient lying on a camp stretcher under a tree. On a couple of occasions, we were collected in a small plane sent up from Nairobi and flown up to the Kenyan Sudanese border to operate on several Sudanese refugees who had crossed the border into Kenya because of the ongoing conflicts happening in their country. Dr Sven, using his expertise, operated on several very complex eye cases. I clearly remember one of these cases: Dr Sven was asked to remove the eye of a small girl whose face had been mauled by a hyena. Her face was badly infected and after the eye was removed, she was flown to Nairobi for further treatment. Dr Sven was a very experienced eye specialist whose skills in this field of medicine were very much appreciated by those patients whose eyes problems he addressed. His ability to remove cataracts even in the most remote clinics gave the patient not only the ability to see again, but also the gift of being able to be a productive member of the community again.

Risk was a constant on any of these medical safaris. On another occasion, Nurse George, a driver and I were heading to our final clinic after two days visiting patients in an isolated part of Kenya. Suddenly, our Land Rover stalled and shuddered to a stop. It was not an ideal place to stop, in the middle of nowhere, with a very temperamental radio. We had food and water, and each other, and that was about all. The road ran through remote country and our chances of seeing another human being were extremely low. The driver, who happened to be a locally trained car mechanic, was trying to sort out the problem, but he wasn't having any luck. So, there we sat. The hours ticked by. Suddenly, we heard a vehicle in the distance coming towards us, making us quite hopeful that help was at hand. Around the corner in a great cloud of dust came a Land Rover. The vehicle screamed to a halt. The driver emerged from the cab. We couldn't believe our eyes. It was a nun, our very own 'flying nun' Sister Jane, and this nun was not your usual nun! Originally from America, this nun was exceptional. She lived in this far-off area, on her own, carrying out basic medical care for the wandering nomads. A very interesting person with a great sense of humour, her stories would keep the world entertained for years. As the red dust settled all over us, she casually greeted us with, 'Hi, what's happened?' We explained our situation and that the vehicle just wouldn't start. She asked a few questions of the driver and then she turned to me and asked, 'What are your plans?' 'Not sure,' I replied. 'Do you have any ideas?' She thought for a few minutes, then she said, 'There are a few Catholic Fathers living in a place about 45 minutes away. Barbara, I could take you there. They have a radio and you could contact Kapedo and let them know what's happened. You guys better stay with the vehicle. It's the back of beyond out here, but you never know who might come along.' I talked with the men and they were happy with that. 'We will carry on working on the vehicle,' they said. So off I went with the flying nun, just about flying along the very rough roads; at times I thought I would be going to heaven sooner rather than later!

We arrived at the Catholic Fathers' compound and the nun jumped out of the vehicle and knocked on the door. After some minutes, an elderly Catholic Father came to the door and listened to Sister Jane as she explained what had happened, and who I was. She asked if I could stay the night in their guest wing. The Father looked at me, smiled and welcomed me into their home. There were four of them living there, all from Ireland. The housekeeper showed me their guest wing, and I was invited to join them for an evening meal at six. Once I had said goodbye to Sister Jane, thanking her for her help, she climbed into her vehicle and off she went, my latest angel, in a cloud of red dust. I enjoyed their cold-water shower immensely, shedding the dirt and the dust of the day, made myself as presentable as I could with the clothes I'd brought along, and just before six I wandered down to the lounge to await dinner. As I walked in, the Father who'd welcomed me invited me to help myself to a cold drink from the fridge in the far corner of the room. I opened the fridge door; what a sight! The fridge was full of soft drinks, beer, wine, and anything else one might fancy. I helped myself to a soft drink and wandered over to meet the other Fathers. They asked me where I was from. When I said I was from New Zealand, the rest of the evening was spent talking rugby. They couldn't believe they were entertaining a girl from New Zealand, the home of the All Blacks. I couldn't believe that in the middle of nowhere was a group of elderly Catholic Fathers who were my hosts for the evening. I asked about using their radio to be informed that it wasn't working. So that was that. No solution to our predicament yet in sight! Although I never did find out what they were doing there, the fact that they were there suited me. I spent a pleasant night and just before six o'clock in the morning there was a knock on my door. When I answered it, there was Nurse George. They had got the vehicle fixed and were ready to take me back to the hospital. After breakfast, I thanked my new friends, jumped into our vehicle and we headed home.

Left to die: A cultural dilemma

Another medical safari I was involved in put me in a very difficult situation. The situation arose through a clash of cultural values and expectations. We had stayed overnight in a small village where we had a basic medical clinic and the next day, were heading even further out for another one. We were in Pokot country, amongst the nomads who wandered this area of Kenya with their cattle. It was mid-morning when we came around a corner to find, lying under a tree, a pile of blankets. This was an unusual sight out there in the middle of nowhere. I asked the driver to stop and he backed up. Nurse George and I got out of the vehicle and walked cautiously over to the pile. George bent down and slowly lifted the top layer. To our shock, there was an old lady lying there, who had a small gourd of water and nothing more. I looked at Nurse George and asked, 'What has happened? Why is she here?' Looking at me, he replied, 'She is a Pokot lady, obviously not able to keep up with the tribe as they moved on.' 'What will happen to her now?' I asked naively, although deep down I already knew the answer. 'She will die here, or she will be killed by hyenas.' 'You're joking!' I declared, but I knew by the look on his face that he was not. 'What do we do now?' I asked him. 'What do you, Sister Barbara, want to do?' he asked. 'I can't leave her here for the hyenas to get. We need to take her with us or take her back and ask those people for help. I couldn't go to bed tonight knowing that she was lying out here. Could you?' 'No,' said Nurse George, 'It's a difficult situation.'

Nurse George spoke to the woman in her own language and then translated her words. She thought she had already died; when she saw a white person, she thought I was an angel; she had never seen a white person before. She went on to tell Nurse George that her tribe had moved on early that morning, as they were looking for feed for their animals. She was willing to be left behind as she couldn't keep up with the others. After some time talking with the woman, we decided to take her with us and head back to the village where we had been staying. Nurse George knew some of the people there and was sure they would be able to assist us. This was a serious cultural dilemma. I felt that what I was doing was right.

What would you have done?

35. Zambia, via Sweden and England

This was now 1990. I had begun to wonder what God had in store for me next. The longer I worked in Kenya the less sure I was about where I would stand with the Provincial Medical Officer of Health should something happen to go wrong. One day Dr Sven mentioned that a Swedish Mission was on the lookout for an experienced nurse to take over from the current Swedish Matron of the Mpwonge 120-bed mission hospital in the copper belt region of Zambia. While in Kenya I flew down to visit the hospital in Zambia, carrying on to England via Sweden, where I met members of the Swedish Mission Board. The interviews went well, and I was planning on heading to Zambia after a few weeks' holiday in the United Kingdom.

However, there were also personal issues I had to deal with. I had continued to suffer frequent and increasingly severe pain each month. Although no-one else knew this, during my time in Kenya I was on constantly high doses of pain relief. I popped pills in private and kept pushing myself in public. So, I took a break and flew to England for some rest but also to visit my gynaecologist there.

A tough decision to be made

I rang the Chelsea Women's Hospital and managed to get an appointment. When I described for the gynaecologist the huge amount of pain relief I was taking, he looked at me and said, 'Barbara you can't keep doing this. You have three choices. If you keep taking the pain relief to be able to carry on working, in a few years' time your kidneys will be in serious trouble and then you will have to face those issues. Secondly, you could head back to New Zealand, where they could monitor you more closely and put you on different medication.' (The medication I'd been on for a few years for the endometriosis had ended up causing me problems, including raising my cholesterol level. Given my family history of heart disease, staying on this medication was not a long-term option.) He continued, 'The third option is to have a total hysterectomy. We will also remove your ovaries so you will be relieved of the severe pain you are experiencing. I would suggest you think about these options and let me know what you decide,' the specialist said. This was a Friday and I said I would get back to him on Monday.

Although this was a long time ago, I still remember walking out of the hospital devastated. The choices were serious, and radical. My mind was racing. I loved working in the developing world. I knew if I went home to New Zealand, I would find it hard to nurse in a different environment from the ones I'd been used to. I was unsure what to do. I was staying with my friend Wendy in London and we talked about the pros and cons. I was only 38 years old; I had no idea what the future would hold regarding marriage and having children. I spent that weekend praying, thinking, and wrestling with my thoughts, my feelings, and my ongoing pain for which I was continuing to take the strong pain relief and the medication for endometriosis. What decision would I make? And what was God saying in all of this? I repeated this last question more than the others.

By the time Monday morning came, I had made my decision. I would go ahead with the total hysterectomy. Once I had recovered, I planned to head to Zambia. I rang the hospital and arranged an appointment for the following day. Tuesday arrived and I saw the specialist, who asked me what I had decided. 'I have decided to go ahead and have the hysterectomy,' I said, my voice trembling. He looked at me and said, 'I realise that it has been a hard decision to come to, but if you want to stay nursing in the developing world you really don't have a choice. It doesn't make the decision any easier though.' I gave him a wee smile, as I held back the tears. 'When would you be able to operate?' I asked hesitantly. 'I have a space on Friday,' was his reply. 'Oh!' I said, 'I guess I was hoping for some more time …' Deep down, however, I knew I was doing the right thing. I summoned my courage. 'Okay,' I said, 'I'll take it.'

My friend Liz, who I had met at Bible College in Tasmania, had flown over from Holland where she was working. On Friday morning, she accompanied me to the hospital, and I was taken to theatre in the afternoon. As they wheeled me along the corridor, I remember shedding tears; tears of relief that there would be no more persistent pain, and tears of anguish for the potential children I would never give birth to.

Having delivered many babies in New Zealand and around the world, this was the hardest fact to confront. What a choice! What a cost! It doesn't get much harder than that.

Wonderfully looked after by my English friends, I recovered well from the surgery. Six weeks later I headed to Zambia along with my new HRT (hormone replacement therapy) medication patch.

36. A Fresh Beginning

When I arrived in Zambia in 1990, I flew into the capital, Lusaka, where I was met by Swedish missionary staff from the Mpongwe Mission Hospital, and driven to Mpongwe, six hours away in the Copperbelt Region. After a long and tiring journey, we arrived at the mission compound. I was taken to my new home, on a quiet, private street away from the main road leading into the hospital. It was wonderful; a lovely two-bedroom house, with a beautiful garden and tennis court.

My new home was part of a cluster of homes, housing one Swedish and two English families. My neighbours were all connected to the hospital, working either in the medical field or in the support roles. My house was rather like a New Zealand house, with running water, an electric stove and a washing machine. The furniture had come from Sweden, and all the linen was supplied, along with a Swedish bike, which I rode around the compound and down to the hospital. To me it was five-star accommodation compared to some of the places I'd lived in. The contrasts between my dust-laden tent in Somalia, and my corrugated tin shed in Ethiopia and this beautifully furnished house in Zambia blew my mind.

The hospital had a mission farm connected to it, fifteen minutes from the hospital. The farm supported the hospital by providing fresh milk, meat and vegetables and was managed by a lovely Swedish couple, Anders and Birgitta, and their three young boys. I became part of their family and they all became a part of mine. Keith, an agricultural economist from the United Kingdom, also lived close by, as he was involved in working with United Kingdom and Zambian government projects. Although he wasn't part of the mission, he was extremely supportive of the work of the hospital and the mission farm and spent time with us all, but especially the farm family and me.

The hospital had 120 beds and was reasonably well equipped with many of the machines and equipment coming directly from Sweden. It had a maternity unit, medical and surgical male and female wards, separate children's wards, a basic laboratory, an operating theatre, a pharmacy, and a kitchen which produced meals for the patients three times a day. Surgery was carried out when a surgeon was available. There was a large workshop, which carried out the all the maintenance on the hospital and in our houses. It employed several local men, who worked alongside the expat plumbers and electricians, and serviced the vehicles we used. We needed these vehicles for daily clinics and for getting supplies from Ndola, the nearby city. Occasionally, we would need a vehicle to drive to Lusaka to collect medicines and other necessities that couldn't be bought locally; a return road trip was over 600 kilometres, which often took over nine hours because of the state of the roads.

The mission hospital was staffed by doctors and nurses, coming at varying times from England, Sweden and New Zealand. Over the years, it had acquired a good reputation for its standard of care, so much so that expatriates from all over Zambia would come and consult with the Swedish doctors to receive treatment. We also had registered Zambian nurses and midwives, a trained Zambian x-ray technician, laboratory staff and a Zambian clinical medical officer. One of the expat doctors also worked as a dentist, which usually meant pulling teeth. (No holes were filled as we didn't have the equipment for doing that.) My role in this mission was to learn the ropes from the current matron of the hospital who was about to go on leave.

Zambian Nurses' Council

As a foreigner wanting to work in their country, I had to submit my nursing and midwifery papers to the Zambian Nurses' Council. They didn't require an interview, but looked at all my papers and my experience, including my extensive midwifery experience in Pakistan. They then agreed to give me Zambian general nurse's registration but not Zambian midwifery registration, as their training course for a midwife was one year, whereas the New Zealand midwifery training I had done lasted six months. I couldn't change their minds despite letters and a phone call, so I quietly carried on supporting the Zambian midwives in our hospital and carrying out the more complex deliveries they did not know how to manage, always supervised by them. It worked well and together we delivered many mothers and babies. Sadly, many of those we delivered were HIV positive, and this was becoming more and more common.

The HIV and AIDS epidemic

I encountered my first HIV positive patients and my first patients with AIDS in Zambia. AIDS, or acquired immune deficiency syndrome, is a chronic, potentially life-threatening condition caused by the human immunodeficiency virus (HIV) damaging the immune system. HIV interferes with the body's ability to fight the organisms that cause disease. In 1990, the numbers of people testing positive for the virus and those dying of AIDS were climbing every day. This situation pre-dated the introduction of anti-retro viral HIV medications. If someone was unlucky enough to be HIV positive in Zambia at that time, life expectancy was two to three years. Orphans were becoming an increasing concern, and money was beginning to be put into education to try and prevent the spread of this condition. The Zambian government was being pressured to acknowledge this situation and act.

Closer to home, at the Mission Hospital, a high percentage of our patients were either HIV positive or had AIDS. With several of our pregnant women HIV positive, there came a new dilemma: should the mother breastfeed? There was strong evidence that the HIV virus could be transmitted through breast milk. But this was Zambia. There was no other option to breastfeeding, as the cost of milk powder formula was beyond the parents' reach. This was one of the many AIDS related issues we encountered daily.

Within the hospital, a high percentage of our adult patients were found to be HIV positive. Many adults who were admitted to the hospital with common complaints would not respond to standard treatments. These patients, after some brief counselling, were offered the quick HIV Du Pont test which could be done in our lab. The result was given to the patient in the afternoon, with more support. I spent many an afternoon with my interpreter Dorothy, informing the patient of the result. This was an extremely sobering job, which had life-changing implications for all involved. Some of these patients, who looked very fit and well but weren't responding to the normal treatment for a complaint such as pneumonia, didn't believe us when their blood test came back HIV positive. It presented challenges medical staff hadn't had to deal with before.

'A new red dress and new shoes; ready to dance for Jesus.'

As the number of patients with HIV grew and those with AIDS also multiplied, we started a home-based programme led by an amazing Zambian nurse called Idah. Twice a week, we would go out and support AIDS patients in their homes, where they were being cared for by their families. We also gave HIV and AIDS education to the family members. I still remember to this day the first home visit I made with Nurse Idah. We arrived at a home, a very basic mud hut with a straw roof. We were invited inside and introduced to a man, his wife and their daughter, who was lying on a grass mat on the floor. (I will call her Jane.) She was terribly sick with AIDS and was not long for this earth. I went over and shook her hand and she said to Nurse Idah, 'I need a red dress.' Nurse Idah translated this for me, and then she asked the daughter, 'Why do you need a red dress?' Jane replied in a very weak voice, 'When I die and go to heaven, I want to have a new red dress to wear for Jesus.' Nurse Idah assured her that we would do our best and would call back in a couple of days with a new red dress. Jane smiled. After talking to the mother and asking how she was coping, and leaving some flour, tea and sugar for the family, we left. A couple of days later we returned and delivered, as promised, a new red dress. When we walked into the hut, despite Jane's increasing weakness, she still reached out her hand and took the dress, held it so tightly, and smiled. She then beckoned Nurse Idah to come closer and said in her own language, 'I need some shoes now.' Nurse Idah burst out laughing and then translated for me, 'Jane wants a pair of shoes.' We all smiled as she shared with us via Nurse Idah's translation, 'She wants to wear her dress and her new shoes and dance with Jesus when she dies.' Jane reached out her hand and held our hands tight, and tears streamed down all our faces. We prayed with her and left, assuring her that we would try hard to find her the shoes she wanted. We went to the market and found a pair of shoes which we thought would probably fit her before calling by the house to drop them off. Jane eyes were glowing; she took the shoes, held them tight, then asked her mother to put them on her feet. The shoes fit her perfectly. We left, saying that we would call by in a couple of days. A few days later we returned as promised. As we pulled up to the gate the mother came to out to greet us, telling Nurse Idah that Jane had passed away a couple of hours after we had left them, and yes, she was wearing her new dress and her new shoes ready to dance with Jesus.

My interpreter

Dorothy was my main interpreter, a lovely lady who had three children. When I did ward rounds, she was always with me and helped me in the clinics in the afternoon. Without her, I would have been lost. One day, I got word from New Zealand that my mother was very ill, and so I flew home to support her and Dad. I was away for six weeks, and when I returned, I didn't see Dorothy. I asked the staff and they said, 'Sister Barbara, come with us.' I walked with them down to the single room where our critically ill patients were always nursed. 'She's in there,' they said, as we approached the door of the room. I opened the door and walked into the room. There, lying on the bed, huddled up in the foetal position, was Dorothy. She was extremely ill and had lost a huge amount of weight. I could hardly recognise her. I reached over and held her hand. After some time, she wearily asked me a question, 'Sister Barbara, do I have AIDS?' I didn't know what to say to this special lady who had become so much a part of my life. 'What do you think?' I put the question back to her, as I struggled to find some words. 'I do have it,' she responded. I reached down and hugged her. For a moment time stood still. 'Yes,' I said, 'I am so sorry.' After a few minutes, she said, 'Can I go home? I want to be with my children. My house is nearby. Do I have to stay here?' 'No,' I said, 'I'm sure you can go home. I'll talk to the doctor and we will arrange it. We can take you in the hospital vehicle.' Her voice trembled as she pleaded with me. 'Sister Barbara, please pray for me and my family. I'm not worried about myself. I'm worried about my children. My husband died of AIDS some time ago and now I am dying. What will happen to my children? Please make sure they know about AIDS.' I reassured her, saying, 'I will.' Taking her hand, I prayed for her, and for her family, realising that her time at home with her family was not going to be long. We arranged to take her home by truck, with a mattress from the hospital.

Dorothy's family and the staff rallied around and nursed her at home. I called twice a day, taking her soup, and spending time just sitting with her, holding her hand and praying for her, as she grew weaker and weaker. A few days later, at a time when I was on duty, a message came to say that she had died. Some members of the staff and I went to spend time with her, to thank God for her life and to support her family. It was a real privilege to be asked to take part in her funeral. The following day, as we all stood around her graveside, I was able to thank God for the life of Dorothy and to pray for her family. Dorothy was such a special lady in my life, and a good friend. I kept my promise; Nurse Idah and I continued to talk to many people about AIDS, including Dorothy's children and her extended family.

A new addition to the hospital

One day, we heard that a very wealthy dentist had died in Italy and his family wanted to donate his fancy dentist's chair, which had all the bells and whistles, to a worthy cause in the developing world. By some miracle the chair arrived at the Mpongwe Mission Hospital, I believe through the actions of someone at the Italian Embassy in Lusaka. The chair was installed in a small room, which became the dental surgery, and one of our expat doctors at the time began pulling teeth for the many Zambian people who were suffering acute and chronic pain from toothache. Although we couldn't drill teeth or put in fillings, our patients were experiencing so much pain that they were happy just to have their aching teeth removed.

Soon after the chair arrived, the English doctor who also worked as a basic dentist, was about to go on leave; he offered to teach me how to pull teeth, and of course I agreed. I was given a crash course in giving local anaesthetic for the pulling of both top and bottom teeth. The doctor also showed me how to dig out the roots of broken teeth which had often been broken and rotten for years. After the doctor went on leave, I started running a clinic a couple of afternoons each week. Many patients coming to this clinic were HIV positive and some even had AIDS. Protection for me was uppermost in my mind; I managed to get hold of a plastic shield attached to a helmet such as a motorbike rider would wear. I always tried to double glove as well, despite sometimes having holes in our recycled specimens. When patients arrived with infected teeth and were in a lot of pain, they were given some pain relief, put on a course of antibiotics and told to return to the clinic a few days later. For those who didn't have an infection, after inserting the anaesthetic in the correct place, I would wait, and then begin to pull the tooth out. Some patients had a mouth full of broken roots which were causing them pain and they would want these roots removed. This condition was much harder to deal with. It took a lot more effort and skill. The relief on their faces once I had completed their requests, and their words of thanks, made all the hard work worthwhile.

However, I was extremely aware of the risk I was taking. Only once did I stop working on a patient's teeth; this man had decided that he didn't want any anaesthetic prior to the procedure and ended up almost biting me. I refused to continue treating him, instead suggesting he get the bus and travel to the nearest hospital, a couple of hours away, and get them to sort his tooth out. It would cost him a lot of money, whereas we provided our dental care for free. I think we both learned a lesson that day! I often think of my dental career in Zambia when I sit in the dentist chair in New Zealand, very grateful that we have dental services available here (despite the cost!).

Stepping up to every challenge

Often during my years working overseas, when there was no one else in the area willing to take the challenge on, I just had to step up and do my best. I often wonder what that night nurse supervisor at Greenlane Hospital, who told me off for inserting a drip into a patient, would say now when I was able to give my first anaesthetic; a question I will never get an answer for.

Whenever we had a surgeon come to stay, we would carry out any major surgeries that were required. Once, a surgeon from Sweden came for a few months and at the time we had two patients who needed surgery. One was an older man whose rotting leg needed to be removed, and the other was a woman who had breast cancer and needed a mastectomy. I asked the surgeon about the type of anaesthetic to be used and he told me it was Ketamine, something I was not familiar with. My experience had been with spinal anaesthetic, and with chloroform and ether. He handed me a book and suggested I read all about ketamine; we were to meet in theatre the next morning, as I was to be his anaesthetist! As you can imagine, I didn't sleep that night, tossing and turning, and reading all about ketamine, which was administered through an intravenous drip. It turned out to be an exhausting day in theatre. We prayed before we started any surgery, and on this day, I believe we had some guidance. One operation had to be cancelled, when the elderly man we were operating on began to go into respiratory arrest. The second operation also proved challenging; the drip had been inserted into the patient's arm tissue rather than the vein, so she wasn't getting enough ketamine during the operation and began to stir. Fortunately, I noticed what was happening and was able to quickly reinsert the intravenous drip to allow the ketamine to flow again, and the operation continued, successfully.

Resuscitating our smallest patients

Some of our expat doctors were able to perform Caesarean sections, which was a great service. Had this service not been available, it would have meant a long trip over dirt roads to the nearest big hospital, nearly two hours' drive away. During these procedures, it was always tense in theatre until the baby was out, when the baby's cry would signal that all was well. On the odd occasion when the baby didn't come out crying, the atmosphere in the theatre would become extremely tense. It was usually me who had to jump in to resuscitate the baby, guided by the surgeon. I had learnt intubation techniques in Pakistan and those skills were often used in Zambia with positive results.

One day the new-born baby wasn't responding to the treatment I was giving her. The doctor, who was busy with the mother said to me, 'Draw up a small amount of adrenaline and inject it straight into her heart.' He confirmed the amount needed and then showed me where to place the needle. He stood over me, watching as I inserted the needle, all the while keeping a close eye on the mother lying on the table. Thank God the baby began to respond. I kept on assisting the baby to breathe, using some resuscitation equipment we had; slowly the infant's colour improved and finally we heard the cry we had been waiting for. How overjoyed we were to hear that wail!

When I trained in New Zealand there were always paediatricians around to help. Here it was different; being in these situations was a steep learning curve and one had to be a quick learner. It certainly wasn't a place for the faint-hearted. But every success was a celebration! As in so many situations in the mission field in Africa, we were 'it.' We had to do what we could with what we had, and our experience, skills and ability to make quick decisions were invaluable.

Premature babies and Kiwi ingenuity

In times of crisis, our lack of basic equipment was of great concern. We did have incubators in the hospital, but they were all broken; as they had come from Sweden, we were unable to get local spare parts. Once again, my Kiwi childhood and practical skills learned in the country came in handy. When I was a child, my friend's Anne's father, Clarrie, a sheep farmer, had kept a box with electric lights on the top. He used to keep new lambs in the box and the lights would keep them warm. I described this warming box to the guys in the workshop, and they came up with a makeshift apparatus which I used in Zambia for our wee prem babies. The smallest premature baby we ever had weighed one kilo at birth, and we managed to look after her in our box. She did very well, with our improvised incubator keeping her warm.

Free time in Mpongwe

Most Saturday nights, Keith and I would go out and spend time with the family at the farm. We enjoyed ourselves immensely and became very close friends with Anders, Birgitta and their three young sons. We would make pizzas and sit around and discuss issues that were of concern to us and listen to the news from the wider world. When working in situations overseas, people rely heavily on the international radio stations. My joy was the BBC World Service. That was my sanity when things became tense in working situations. The reporters were like my friends, as I had met quite a few of them when I was working in other parts of Africa, and I enjoyed listening to them in Zambia. I think we all needed those nights around the radio, to connect to each other, but also to the wider world, far away as we were from our own homes.

Another pastime that helped to keep life well-rounded was golf, a game I've always been keen on. I guess I inherited this love of the game from my parents and grandparents. I was never any good at it, but I enjoyed just getting out and walking around and hitting a small white ball. It was a freedom and a time of relaxation that I enjoyed enormously. The nearest golf course was about one hour away from the hospital, and as Keith played golf as well, we would often take off early Saturday morning and go and play a round. After a few weeks, the secretary of the Luanshya Golf Club suggested we seek full membership of the club. For this we would need to fill out a membership application form. Thinking this would be a good option for us we completed our forms and posted them off to the club. Sometime later we received a letter informing us of a time for our interview to see if we would be suitable members. We drove into the town one afternoon and went to the golf club, where we were shown into the president's office and invited to sit down. Introductions were exchanged and he then asked us why we wanted to join the club. We both said, 'To play golf.' At that point he interrupted and said, 'I hope it isn't to drink beer.' Surprised by the question, we both assured him that it wasn't! He stated that many people joined the club just to drink beer and that was not to be encouraged. We told him again that we lived one hour away from the club and would be joining to play golf! He then stood up, shook our hands and welcomed us to the club. We thanked him and left, both commenting in the car on the way home that the interview was certainly different from what we'd been expecting! Over the next two years, we enjoyed golf regularly, and I was fortunate enough to have an English friend, Pat, a keen golfer, come to stay. We had some special times playing golf both in Zambia and later in Zimbabwe.

Family, friends and God

During my time in Zambia, I had many people come to stay, including friends from New Zealand and England, and my Aunty Philippa Swanson from New Zealand. It was wonderful to be able to show them around and introduce them to my new friends, and for them to see the work that was going on at the hospital, as well as in the mobile clinics. I was also able to take them to some of the game parks, and of course, to Victoria Falls, which was a highlight. Their interest, and their companionship, helped to ease my sense of isolation.

To care for myself spiritually, I attended a local church on the compound and was also invited to speak at churches around the town of Mpongwe. A local man, a keen Christian, was willing to translate. The Swedish farm family also provided great spiritual support and letters from friends assuring me of their prayers were always welcome. There were times, however, when the going was tough and I felt isolated, especially at times like Christmas, when I knew my family would be gathering to celebrate. At times like this I had many conversations with God. These encounters also helped to ease my loneliness.

Back to the classroom

During this time, I had many long conversations with my friend Keith regarding my future. He was encouraging me to go and get more qualifications, especially if I planned to stay in the relief and development arena. I couldn't really see myself working in a hospital in New Zealand; I thought I would have trouble keeping within the rules and regulations of both the Midwifery and Nursing Councils. My experience in the various situations I'd been working in had taken me out of the nursing arena into work more akin to that of a medical registrar. Keith and I talked long and hard about the possibilities, including course options. I needed to look at a course that would capture and hold my interest as I knew that study itself would be a huge barrier to overcome, not to mention the costs of the course. I'd heard about the master's degree course in Medical Anthropology offered by Brunel University in London. Having struggled at school with reading and writing, I knew that to do such a course would be for me an almost impossible mountain to climb. At the same time, something attracted me to the course, and I knew I needed to find out more about it.

I had a couple of weeks' holiday in England coming up, so while there I went and saw the people at Brunel University and spoke in some depth to them. I was somewhat shattered to discover how much the course would cost. It was going to be around NZ$26,000. On top of that would be the living costs. I mentioned my dyslexia and how I have always struggled to read and that it was still not one of my favourite pastimes. I also informed them that I didn't have a first degree and wondered if I was dreaming to think of starting university study at master's level. Yet, as I shared my story with them, and even though my academic record was hardly brilliant, they were keen for me to join the course. They agreed that it would be a challenge, but said, 'Barbara, you seem to be someone who relishes a challenge.'

I spoke with friends. They were all positive, although my parents were a bit concerned about my ability to complete the course. The main stumbling block was going to be the costs of the course and the accommodation. I certainly didn't have the money; the organizations I had been working with didn't pay aid workers a huge amount, unlike some of the bigger agencies on the relief and development scene. If I really wanted to do this, I had to come up with a plan. I approached World Vision New Zealand. They most generously awarded me a scholarship which covered a large percentage of my fees. Friends from around the world made donations as well. With this support, and some of my personal savings, I managed to get the money together that was needed to cover the costs. I'd been unsettled about my future, but now the course in England had become a real possibility. It would be starting in the middle of the year and I would need somewhere to work in the intervening months.

Moving on

Over the coming weeks, I spent time in prayer, asking God for clear direction regarding my future. I felt God was leading me out of Zambia into something new. Things in Mpongwe were also changing; the Swedish Free Baptist mission had decided to review the whole work of the mission, looking in some depth at the work, and the staff. There would be upheavals. With my contract nearing completion, it was clearly time for me to move on. Though my time in Zambia was coming to an end, my experience nursing patients with HIV and AIDS was to prove beneficial to the next part of my missionary journey, in yet another part of Africa.

37. Tanzania

A serious situation in Tanzania was impacting every aspect of life – and death. Increasing numbers of people were being infected with the HIV virus. Concerns were growing about the effects of this epidemic on the people, on their cultural practices, on the economy of this largely coffee-producing Bukoba region, and on the increasing number of children orphaned because of AIDS. The local hospital was struggling to cope, faced with a huge influx of patients and severely limited treatment options, with their medical supplies frequently running out. Many families of patients diagnosed with AIDS wouldn't even take them to the hospital, knowing it was hopeless to expect any treatment. Many just didn't have the money to pay the hospital's admission fee. What's more, if they did take their loved one to hospital and the person died there, these families were immediately faced with the challenge of getting the body home again which was not easy in a country like Tanzania. Many of those who owned pickup trucks would charge large amounts of money to take the deceased back to their village. This was an unaffordable practice for most people, but taking the body back to the deceased village was customary practice in Tanzania, and an important one. There you could be buried, and only there your soul could rest in peace. You can imagine their anguish.

This was the situation when I arrived in Tanzania at the start of 1993, as a result of a meeting with the Director of World Vision in Tanzania, Bruce McConchie, a friend of mine and a fellow New Zealander. Alert to the growing crisis in that country, he was keen to start up an HIV/AIDS program. Knowing I had been involved in setting up HIV/AIDS programs in Zambia, he was keen for me to come and join his team in Tanzania. It suited me perfectly, as I had a nine-month window before I was due in England in September to start my degree course. As part of the degree, I had to undertake some field research, so the move to Tanzania was ideal; I envisaged undertaking some research there. It also gave me an opportunity to work closely with local staff, who taught me so much.

So there I was in Tanzania, I'd been assigned to work in the Kagera Region of Tanzania, and I was going to be living in Bukoba a city of over 80,000 which was on the shores of Lake Victoria. Surrounding Bukoba were many coffee and banana plantations. Much of World Vision's work was in the many villages and we had daily reminders of the reason for our being there. Often, when we were out visiting patients who were being nursed at home, we would drive past men on bicycles, each with a large parcel strapped to the bike rack. This parcel would be wrapped up in banana leaves and tied tightly to the bike; I soon learnt that each parcel contained a deceased person who was being returned home, possibly having died in a hospital or clinic, likely from AIDS. It was sobering.

Our work

Working with an amazing Tanzanian nurse called Mary and other local staff, we began to plan how we could assist in some small way to deal with the enormous impact of AIDS. Our planning was made easier because World Vision had been working in this area for some time and was already well known for its efforts. However, I would learn that there were certain protocols to be followed; mostly, many meetings would be held, sometimes lasting for hours, and we would listen to what was being said by the elders. Sometimes, the meetings would go on for most of the day. 'It is all about relationships, beginning by building trust and respect,' Mary told me. It all took time, and it was certainly time well spent. HIV/AIDS was changing life in the villages like nothing had before, and the leaders of the community had to consider their guidance carefully. Not only was there a huge stigma about HIV/AIDS, with no-one wanting to talk openly about it, but there were also huge numbers affected, seemingly more every day. Most people in the area knew someone who had the virus or were supporting family members looking after AIDS orphans. Many were also struggling with a positive diagnosis themselves. During those years before anti-retroviral drugs, being diagnosed HIV positive was effectively a death sentence. With such an enormous challenge, it was important to be well-informed and to plan our strategy as sensitively as we could.

Daunting as it was, we had to start somewhere. After discussing all viewpoints, the team decided it would be best to start small, in villages where World Vision had been working, because relationships had already been established there. A meeting with the leaders was held to talk about our proposal. Then, the leaders invited the community to gather, and the talk began. Working with the community, a plan was developed. The strategy would include: support packages for patients who were being nursed at home as well as for the family members caring for them; a community education programme about HIV/AIDS and how it is spread; and the training of local people selected by the community who would, once trained, become educators and counsellors.

We received funding from a couple in New Zealand for this programme; an amazingly generous and timely gift. Working closely with the community leaders, we started our plan, and gradually, over some weeks, people began to talk more openly about what was happening in their families and in their community. Meanwhile, this epidemic was growing at an alarming rate. Despite the fear and the folklore stories that persisted, the community began to open up and share what was happening with one another. There were lots of stories and myths as to how HIV and AIDS were brought to the region and by whom. Some people said it came from Uganda, during a conflict a few years earlier, some said the virus was put into the condoms which were flooding into Tanzania at the time from the west. The stories weren't helpful. One day a village elder stood up at a meeting and said, 'When a snake comes into the house, no one asks where that snake came from; the snake is killed. No one knows where this HIV/AIDS problem came from. The point is, it is here, and we need to stop it from spreading and support those who have got HIV and those who have AIDS.' Wise words from a wise man.

Community members also chose candidates to be trained in HIV/AIDS education and basic counselling skills. My co-worker Mary was brilliant; being a local, she had standing in the community, and was able to get the message across. The teaching took different forms, including discussions, lectures, role-plays and lots of singing. Over time, as trust and confidence grew, the trainees slowly began to share their stories, their fears, and their concerns.

Mary and I spent much of our time visiting AIDS patients in their homes. Thanks to the funding from generous New Zealanders, we were able to provide food items for the patients and their families; it wasn't much, but it was something. Many families managed to provide truly amazing care for their dying family member, even while their loved ones lay on beds made only of banana leaves on mud floors in simple huts. With very little, they provided the love and support that was needed. Many accepted that their care was not just going to be needed for this loved one who was dying. They would need to care for many more family members who would sadly follow the same path; the path that they too might find themselves on.

Unlike other illnesses that strike the elderly, the infirm and children, HIV/AIDS hit people in the prime of their lives, which had an unprecedented impact; the rise in the number of children orphaned through AIDS was alarming. Many were already traumatized by having seen both parents die. Then, barely in their teens, they had become the main caregivers for their siblings, first supporting their mothers as they nursed their fathers, and then nursing the mothers as they lay dying. They had been robbed of their childhood. Also, because it was considered more important to educate the son rather than the daughter, invariably the young girls were taken out of school to care for family members and robbed of their education. The flow on effects of all of this would change these communities for generations.

One day, when visiting a village, we were asked by the leader to call in to see a man who was extremely ill. We walked up the overgrown path to his hut, where Mary knocked on the partially open door. There was no reply. So, she knocked again, calling out to see if anyone was at home. A young girl, maybe six years old, appeared at the door. She signalled for us to come in. Mary led, and I followed her into the hut. As we entered, we noticed a wee toddler sitting silently in the corner. Lying on the floor was a young man. He was very ill, and we could see that he was dying; he was extremely weak and could hardly speak. We approached him and Mary knelt to speak with him. Slowly, he told us that he was dying. His wife had departed this life a few days earlier. He was alone with his two small children. He mentioned a neighbour who regularly called in, but she was also caring for her own family members. His main caregiver was his young daughter. He told us he just wanted to stay here; this was his home. He knew he was dying. He hoped the neighbour would look after his children. It was a tragic situation. As we sat in this man's hut that day, the horrendous reality of the HIV virus hit us hard. We spoke to his neighbour, who said she would continue to keep an eye on him. We gave her supplies to assist in caring for this man. A few days later we heard that the young man had died, and the neighbour was looking after his two small children. How long that arrangement would last, we couldn't say, given the ravages of the disease in that community. How different things would have been for him and his family if he had been born in New Zealand.

Graduation of our trained HIV/AIDS educators and counsellors

After weeks of training, the graduation day for our trained HIV/AIDS educators and counsellors arrived. What excitement there was! The new graduates were each presented with a bicycle to assist them in their work. These bicycles, funded by our kind supporters from New Zealand, were real assets, not only to the workers, but also to the community. They were used for many purposes; carrying supplies from the market, transporting the workers out to the remote villages to spread the HIV/AIDS education message, and visiting AIDS patients being cared for in their homes. Bicycles were also vital in transporting patients to and from the health clinics. Happily, the home-based care counselling programme continued to grow. Over the years that followed, the number of people trained in this programme increased sufficiently to begin to make an impact.

The robbery

When I was assigned to work in Bukoba, I had an agreement that I would take a break in Arusha at the end of every eight-week stint. I would fly down to Arusha and stay with my Kiwi hosts, Bruce McConchie, his wife Margaret and their two children, whose hospitality I really appreciated. In return I was able to bring them fresh fish from Lake Victoria, which they loved. One day, after returning from a weekend in Arusha, I arrived back at my room to find the door open. Horrified, I saw that the room had been totally trashed. Most of my belongings had been taken, including my clothes, books, papers, my gumboots and, most importantly, my food. The little I owned in the world had disappeared. I was devastated. My Tanzanian colleagues were very upset that this had happened and were very supportive, helping me out with the things I needed. I contacted Bruce, my boss in Arusha, to explain what had happened. He needed to know, and suggested I contact my insurance company in London.

I rang my insurance company in England, taking some time to make the connection. They asked that I go to the police station and report the robbery, and then send them the receipts for what I'd lost. I patiently explained to them that I was in a remote part of Tanzania, and I didn't have any receipts for my belongings. I told them I couldn't supply the information they were requesting. I informed them that I would go to the local police station and see if I could get a report that would provide the necessary paperwork. A Tanzanian colleague, John, accompanied me to the local police station where we were told to go around the back of the station, to a small office. There I would be able to explain what had happened. As we walked around the back of the police station, we came across a large group of prisoners sitting on the ground. A couple of guards were standing over them, each with a large stick. Just as we approached one of the guards lifted his stick and was about to strike the prisoners. The prisoners all turned suddenly and looked at us. On seeing us the guard quickly lowered his stick. Being one of only a few white people in Bukoba at that time meant that I was used to being stared at wherever I went. I was shown into the office and with the help of my colleague, I completed the paperwork. I was told to call back in a few days' time to collect the report, which I duly did.

Once I had the report, I sent everything off to the insurance company in England. Some months later I received a small payment for the items that had been stolen. As I went around the place in the weeks after the robbery, I was on the lookout for my stolen goods, but I never found any of the items. As we were very close to the Ugandan border, the items may have been taken there. Being robbed at any time is an unsettling experience; to be robbed in a foreign country was even harder. I was certainly left feeling very unsettled and incredibly nervous; I was so thankful I hadn't been there when the robbery took place.

University, here I come!

Although somewhat shaken, I had to leave this unsettling experience behind and concentrate on what was ahead – University! As the time came for me to leave Bukoba, and Tanzania, I went to see the Bukoba Provincial Medical Officer of Health and spoke to him about the master's course I was about to undertake in England. I asked him if he was willing for me to come and do some of the research in his area. He agreed. He was very supportive and wished me all the best for my studies. Knowing I would return to the country, I left Tanzania on a Wednesday and started at Brunel University in London a week later. It was September 1993, and it was to be a huge culture shock.

As my study programme in England had been all arranged, I had no trouble getting into the United Kingdom as a student; I had official letters from London's Brunel University, where I was enrolled to complete a one-year master's degree in Medical Anthropology. Initially, I lived in the halls of residence at the university but after a couple of weeks I had had enough. A few young students thought it would be a great laugh to cook their bacon and eggs at 3.00 am and deliberately burn them, which set off the fire alarm, with the inevitable arrival of fire engines, their sirens piercing the night air. Naturally the halls had to be evacuated. Standing outside in my slippers, wrapped up in my dressing gown at 3.00 am was not what I had expected, and this was not what I'd come to University for. Fortunately, I had a friend, Wendy, living near the university who agreed to take me as a boarder, and I caught the local bus to travel to Brunel to attend my lectures.

The cultural shock of living in England surprised me. I had to adapt to so many different aspects of life and had so much to learn, which was quite painful at times. I'd come from a remote town in Tanzania to one of the world's busiest cities, and that was a huge adjustment. On top of that, starting university study was daunting enough, without having to learn all about computers, which I hadn't even seen before. At times I felt like I'd arrived from another planet. I had some comfort though. Many other students in my class were mature students like me, and I could see I wasn't the only one struggling to survive in those early days.

I tried hard to get my head around the workings of the computer. After I was shown what to do three times, my teacher, an incredibly patient librarian, finally asked me, 'Barbara, where do you come from?' I explained to her that I was originally from New Zealand, but that for some years I had been working in remote places in the developing world, where computers were not yet part of the scene! She was kind enough to help, and eventually I got the knack of using these things to do my work, which was huge.

Despite all my training and the nursing and midwifery qualifications I had gained, completing a master's degree in one year was a big stretch. We were required to do a lot of reading, write numerous assignments, and attend a programme of regular tutorials. The lecturers were extremely helpful, guiding us through the preparation required for the first of our many essays; I wrote mine and duly submitted it to the course professor. He marked it and wrote across the top, 'You need to write like an anthropologist rather than a nurse.' That was hard for me to do. The workload was heavy and at times I struggled, wondering if I had made the right choice. Having wrestled with reading all my life, I found the reading requirements for the course daunting, at times overwhelming, but I was determined to succeed, so I became sharply focused. As the months went on, I managed to do well in my assignments, and this gave me the impetus to work even harder. My years of experience working in the developing world gave me examples I could use to illustrate the points I was trying to make as I wrote my essays. Caught up as I was in the unrelenting pace of the course programme, I didn't have much time to myself to enjoy London.

As part of my course of study, I continued preparing for my research project, which was to take place in Tanzania, including spending many hours discussing the focus of my research with my tutor. Eventually, I decided to focus on the impact of HIV/AIDS on cultural practices, narrowing the scope to the villages I had been working in immediately prior to coming to England. This fitted well within the discipline of Medical Anthropology. I was indebted to Paul Farmer, a well-known medical anthropologist, whose work in Haiti gave me additional insight into the impacts of HIV/AIDS on local populations. I completed all the assignments, which included several essays, and then I began to work on the final preparation for my field work, which would be followed by the submission of the thesis and the exams. The next few months were going to be intense.

Soon afterwards, I flew off to Tanzania and caught the flight to Bukoba. I booked into a local hostel which was run by the Lutheran church. This was my home for the next three months. I caught up with my former Tanzanian colleagues and they updated me on what they had been doing over the time that I had been away. I also shared with them what my plans were for the coming months, including the survey I was planning to conduct. I was extremely grateful to the World Vision staff, who assisted me in so many ways while I was with them. Without their support, I would not have been able to achieve what I did.

As part of my research, my colleague Mary and I would spend hours in the villages, sitting and listening to locals as they shared stories about the huge impact AIDS had had, and was continuing to have, on their lives. It was very humbling hearing stories from the wives of men who had died of AIDS, and how they were now having to cope with the disease themselves. They told us how they were forced to pull their children out of school and how their daughters now had to care for their mothers. Some people we interviewed were women in the final stages of life, being cared for by their children. From one woman we learned how culturally unacceptable it was for young children to have to clean up after their parents following severe bouts of diarrhoea and vomiting. In some villages we interviewed families headed by children, where children as young as twelve oversaw their siblings, following the AIDS-induced deaths of their parents. These were not big villages. Prior to AIDS, the number of people dying in the village was around one to two per month. Since the arrival of AIDS, the death toll could be as high as three or four per week, impacting everyone in the village and upsetting the normal routines and patterns of everyday life.

One young girl's story stays with me: She was twelve years old. Her father had died of AIDS and her mother had also contracted the disease. The girl was pulled out of school and nursed her mother until her mother died. She was left with her three brothers to care for. Two days before we visited her in her village, her youngest brother had died of malaria, leaving her with her two younger brothers, who would have been nine and seven years old. She was doing her utmost to provide money so they could go to school and was having an even harder time getting enough food for the table. She told us that some of the men in the village had come to see her, individually. They had offered to help her, but only if she was willing to sleep with them. What a dilemma for a twelve-year-old! She was caught between wanting to keep her wee family together, her responsibility to provide food for them, and her desire to keep her brothers at school. Yet she also knew that if she agreed to take up the offer from the men the chances of her getting AIDS was extremely high. Then who would look after her brothers? Some of her relatives, who lived many miles away, had encouraged her to leave the area and go and live with them. She just didn't want to leave her house, and her family's piece of land. Sadly, she was not the only young girl with such a story.

Another woman had lost her husband to AIDS. She herself had also contracted AIDS. She was struggling to survive, as were her three small children. She knew she was dying and described what normally happened culturally when someone in the village died; ordinarily, everyone would come and bring food for the grieving family. Just before our visit, she'd heard that another villager had died, and the village leaders had asked people to bring food to that grieving family. She was desperate. All she had was a small bunch of bananas. She had nothing else. If she gave the bananas to the grieving family as her contribution, what would her children eat? Yet if she didn't contribute to the grieving family, then when she herself came to die, the village might not offer practical support to her children.

It was clear that these villagers were not only dealing with the devastating effects of AIDS on their lives and families; they also had to face the impact the disease was having on their many traditional customs and way of life; when a person died, for example, the family members were all accustomed to shaving their heads as a mark of respect. This practice signalled to people coming into the village that a family had suffered bereavement, so the visitors would know to offer their condolences. Because of the increasing number of deaths in each village, the practice of shaving their heads stopped. Not only would the whole village have been obliged to have shaved heads but using only a few razor blades to shave the heads of a whole village was also a risky business; some of the people's heads could be cut while being shaved, exposing them to AIDS.

The impact was perhaps hardest on the carers. One day, when we were visiting a remote village, a woman explained to Mary and me how in the past, when someone in her family was sick, she would care for them and they would normally recover. Occasionally they would die. Now, with AIDS, she said, 'You care for people, and they all die. No-one recovers. It's hard, so hard. Usually, the reward for caring for a family member is recovery. With AIDS, it is death.' Because of this disruption to the normal way of things, and the numbers involved, the disturbances to their customary way of life were hitting them hard. Another impact had to do with simple lack of resources; it was customary for villagers to assist the grieving family for several months. Once AIDS took hold, most villagers were devoted to supporting their own grieving families, which didn't leave them the time or energy to support the wider community.

We could see that villagers were grieving not only for the loss of their loved ones. They were also grieving for the loss of their traditional way of life, with its regular routines and social practices that everyone understood. The enormity of the AIDS epidemic forced them to make choices for their own and their family's survival that frequently ran counter to their normal cultural practices, causing them immense mental stress and cultural unease. Along with the physical ravages caused by the disease and the death of the people, AIDS was also destroying traditional village life as they had known it. Nothing was the same anymore. There was no security left and the future was uncertain.

Rwanda

While I was in Tanzania completing this fieldwork, even more disruption was happening in neighbouring Rwanda. A massacre was unfolding between the Hutu and Tutsi. There had been a long history of conflicts between these two groups of people, and in 1994 the ensuing massacre resulted in thousands of Rwandan refugees pouring across the border into Tanzania. Huge refugee camps were set up and World Vision staff were involved in assisting in these camps.

One day the opportunity arose for me to visit the largest refugee camp, Benaco, which by then contained over 850,000 people. We arrived at the camp and drove through it, passing hundreds and hundreds of UNHCR blue plastic shelters. Thousands of people were streaming into the camp, carrying everything they owned on their heads. Devastated men, women and children of all ages, having witnessed horrendous atrocities, walked from the fields of slaughter and despair to cross over the bridge which separated Rwanda and Tanzania. Young, elderly, fragile, pregnant, exhausted, they arrived, shocked and overwhelmed. Now they were safe.

Why God, why?

We headed down to the bridge that formed the border crossing. We were stopped there by the Tanzanian border guards, who asked who we were. The Tanzanian staff explained that they were from World Vision, and the guards pointed to a car park area nearby, telling us to park there. We got out of the vehicle and walked down towards the bridge, passing hundreds of people who were walking in silence, shell-shocked, stunned, some in tears, some with no more tears to shed, traumatized humanity. Words cannot really convey what I witnessed that day. I didn't know any of them, but the fear I could see in their eyes hit me, a fellow human being. Silently, I cried out to God.

With one of the World Vision staff members I walked quietly onto the bridge. We stopped in the middle. Looking over the side of the bridge into the water below, I began to comprehend the horrors of this unfolding situation.

Purple Hands

As I stood silently on the bridge that day, I saw, floating down the Kagera River, six bodies tied together. These were people who had been killed. It was a horrifying sight, a horror I will never forget. That day as I watched them walking across the bridge, I saw the pain in the faces of the people escaping from Rwanda. I stood in silence, just looking into the river. No words could explain the scene. As we stood there that day, I had a heartfelt conversation with God. 'How could this happen?' I asked. 'Why did it happen?' Still not uttering a word, I continued to cry out to God. I felt God responding, and words came into my mind, 'I hear your sadness. Imagine how I am feeling.' With that, a beautiful rainbow appeared in the sky, stretching from Tanzania across the river into Rwanda.

The appearance of the rainbow reminded me that God was present there that day. His heart was broken. His tears were flowing, as were mine, together with the survivors streaming out of Rwanda. I looked back into the river then and saw something jammed between the rocks. It was a young child's naked body. My first reaction was to climb down and bring this wee body back up to the camp where we could arrange for this tiny person to be buried. My Tanzanian colleague held me back, saying, 'Barbara, you can't. You just have to leave the child.' He told me that for the three days the previous week, when the team had been there, there had been so many bodies floating down the river that the water couldn't flow. It's said that over 40,000 bodies floated down the Kagera River into Lake Victoria during those horrendous months when the massacre took place. I could not even begin to imagine what the people of Rwanda had suffered. Later that day we drove back to Bukoba. We travelled in silence, mulling over what we had seen, with deep sadness in our hearts at what had happened, and was still happening, in Rwanda. Aid agencies were there, responding to this huge, unfolding humanitarian disaster. I desperately wanted to get involved then and there, helping where I could, but I knew I was committed to my research. It was heart-wrenching to have to drive away.

Years later, I happened to be in Rwanda where I spent several hours in the Genocide Museum in Kigali, where a friend of mine was working. As I walked in silence through this special place, reading the poignant stories of those who had lost their lives on both sides of the conflict I was moved to tears. As I walked out of the museum, on the wall before me was a blackboard with these words written on it: 'Where will the next massacre be?' Sadly, since then, there have been massacres in many places around the world. Even today, as I write this memoir, they continue to occur.

Traditional healers

I returned to Bukoba to continue my work. During this research phase in Tanzania, I spent time with some of the local traditional healers. These healers were increasingly being used to provide traditional medicine for HIV and AIDS patients, as at the time there were no western medicines that would provide a cure for the disease. Many families with members afflicted with AIDS were already struggling to make ends meet. They didn't have the means to buy the antibiotics and other treatments which might have relieved some of their loved ones' symptoms. Prior to AIDS, the traditional healers didn't charge a fee in monetary terms, but after receiving treatment, the patient or the family gave a gift in kind, which might be a chicken, or some bananas.

Because of the tragedy that was HIV/AIDS, charlatan traditional healers flocked to this afflicted region of Tanzania, setting up their clinics, and offering all sorts of medicines and potions which they said would cure anything and everything, for outrageous prices. Many families, in their desperation to have their son or daughter cured of AIDS, spent the little they had on these miracle cures which, sadly, didn't work.

Later, I spent ten days sitting alongside a more reputable traditional healer in a clinic at the regional hospital in Bukoba. My colleague Mary was there with me. The healer sat behind a large desk and had in front of him a great display of bottles of all shapes and sizes, each filled with liquid. He also had small packets of different leaves and berries. Each patient who came to see him was asked questions pertaining to their whole being. Finally, they were asked about their physical symptoms. Depending on what they said, they were given either a bottle of liquid or a packet of leaves together with instructions on how to drink it, or apply the leaves and berries mixed in water to their rashes. At the end of each day, the traditional healer would take time to speak with me regarding his beliefs and his medicines. One day, I commented that most of the liquid in the bottles and the packets of leaves and berries all looked very similar, and yet the patients coming in to visit him all had different symptoms. I was surprised when he told me that all his treatments were the same, and the liquid or leaves would do the job as required. He went on to say, 'You could take a sample of my treatments and send them to

America and get them tested. They would come back stating some of the components, but they wouldn't be able to measure the psychological component, the belief component.'

The patients came to the traditional healer in faith that he would be able to help them. Indeed, some of the patients returned and Mary and I were able to ask them if the medicines they'd received had made a difference. Many said, 'My diarrhoea stopped. The rash I had disappeared after a few days of applying the leaf and berry medicine.' Sure, they were still HIV positive, or had AIDS. Yet they had a belief in the medicine they had received, and they also had faith in the traditional healer. In that way the medicine had helped them, at least for a while.

'Barbara, they want to circumcise you.'

After my two months in Bukoba, having gained enough information for the research part of my thesis, I left to stay with Bruce and his family in Arusha. There I was able to spend time with some of the Masai tribes who lived nearby. Wonderfully assisted by Tanzanian staff, I spent time in the villages, listening to some of the elders and the traditional birth attendants as they discussed ways they could adapt their traditional cultural practices, which were deemed to be helping the spread of the HIV virus. This included discussing the widespread practice of both male and female circumcision.

One morning Eugenie, my friend and interpreter, and I sat with a group of traditional birth attendants who, in graphic detail, explained to me the whole process of female circumcision, and what they were doing to make the practice safer for the person being circumcised in the light of the HIV/AIDS situation. I had first come across the cultural practice of female circumcision while I was working in Somalia some years before, but that was prior to HIV/AIDS. They were more than happy to answer my questions and I was enormously grateful for their willingness to share. As the conversation ended, they began looking at me, then talking quietly to each other. I was beginning to feel somewhat uncomfortable. I asked Eugenie what was happening, although I suspected I knew what her answer would be before I had even finished asking her the question. 'They want to know if you have been circumcised. If you haven't, they would be willing to do it for you,' she responded with a smile. Part of me was shocked, but the other part wasn't. I very quickly signalled a definite 'No!' and stood up. Crossing my legs, I jumped out of the hut and into the freedom outside. They followed me out, laughing, as did Eugenie. I thanked them for the kind offer, and we said goodbye. Off I went, vastly relieved at my escape.

Later that afternoon, after I'd caught up with some of the other Masai leaders who had agreed to speak with me, we happened to come across my two 'friends' from the morning. They pointed, whispered to each other, and then began to laugh. I responded immediately by crossing my legs and jumping forward, laughing. Many of those around me, watching, burst out laughing as well, joining in the merriment.

38. More Challenges to Come

My time in Tanzania had come to an end. With my return to England, the serious work of writing up all the data I had collected for my thesis began. It was an insanely busy few months. The work was intense. I met regularly with my tutor. We discussed in depth my work for the thesis, and I continued with my writing. The time came for me to sit my exams. As I was doing three different topics for my degree courses, I had three full days of exams where I was required to choose different topics and write an essay on each one. Because of my dyslexia, the University had generously offered me a writer to assist me in the exams, but I said I would be fine. I thought the exams went well. The following week, I submitted the final draft of my thesis to my tutor. I was stunned when she came back saying that she had grave doubts about my whole thesis. She wondered if what I had written had any content from a medical anthropology slant.

She strongly recommended that I re-write it. I couldn't believe my ears! The thesis was due to be submitted to the University two weeks later and I knew I couldn't re-write it in that time. I was extremely upset. I'd met regularly with my tutor following my return to England from Tanzania; she was aware of what my plans were. I didn't know what to do. Doubts came into my mind and I feared letting the people down who'd believed in me, who'd given me scholarships and funding for the course. What was I to do?

I turned to some trusted friends, who were most encouraging. They suggested that I should go with my gut feeling. I strongly believed I'd done my best and was happy with what I'd written. I thought long and hard about this difficult situation I was in. I talked with God and prayed hard before coming to a decision. I would read the thesis through, and maybe make a few alterations. I most certainly was not going to rewrite it. I didn't have the time. Two days before the thesis was due for submission, I got it bound, took it to the University, and handed it in. I walked out of the university, knowing I had done my best. Now the wait for the results of the thesis and the exams would begin.

Return to Tanzania – HIV/AIDS Consultant for World Vision

With my exams behind me and my thesis submitted, I headed back to Tanzania. This time it would be to Arusha, at the base of volcanic Mt. Meru, 100 kilometres southwest of Africa's highest peak, the 5,895 metre Mt. Kilimanjaro, and a gateway to safari destinations. To the west lies Serengeti National Park, home to such wildlife as lions, rhinoceroses, giraffes and leopards, and my favourite, the wart hog, with annual migrations featuring huge herds of wildebeests crossing its plains. I stayed again with Bruce, the World Vision Tanzanian director, his wife Margaret and their children, who were wonderful hosts, until a house became available for me; a cottage attached to a local safari business. Bruce and Margaret gave me a hand moving in and helped me with furnishing the house, for which I was very grateful. My new role was to be HIV/AIDS Co-ordinator. I enjoyed working alongside my Tanzanian colleagues, who taught me so much, trying to find ways to work more effectively with communities to address the ongoing HIV/AIDS issues.

Family visit

I was thrilled when, in 1995, my brother Phil and his wife Christine Best-Walker came to stay. It was wonderful to take them on safari across the Serengeti, and we were fortunate to have two other friends join us, Alistair and Maureen. I had met them when they were part of a New Zealand TV crew, along with kiwi TV personality Judy Bailey, who filmed some of the World Vision work in the Bukoba area. During Phil and Christine's visit, we were honoured to be invited to stay overnight in a Masai boma (village). I was very grateful to Eugenie, my World Vision friend, who came with us, as well as a Masai colleague, Ruth, who guided us through the night's entertainment, which included eating a very raw goat that was killed in Phil's honour, and then joining the Masai for an evening of dancing.

The truck drivers and the prostitutes

Another very important area of the World Vision's HIV/AIDS programme was educating the truck drivers and prostitutes. In those days, no trucks were allowed on the road after sunset; that was the ruling. Consequently, trucking stops had been established along the main route, which began in Dar Es Salaam in the east of Tanzania and ran right across to the west of the country to the Rwandan and Ugandan borders. The truck drivers and their helpers, usually one or two guys, would park at these stops for the night. Small hotels, bars, and basic shops were set up to cater for the truckers. Over time these truck stops spread all along the route and it wasn't long before they had become the size of small villages.

Some of these stops would have as many as sixty to eighty trucks parked up overnight. Quiet during the day, they would become a hub of activity once evening came. Girls and women were hired to work in the hotels and bars, and inevitably many were drawn into prostitution, an ever-increasing business. These stops became a focus for our HIV/AIDS awareness campaign. As part of the education programme, a group of us would sit in the bars and hotels at night. There we would listen to the stories of the women and the truck drivers. The Tanzanian staff would also give simple talks about the HIV/AIDS virus and the risks involved in such an environment.

At the same time, we, along with local leaders, were investigating the possibility of starting income-generating businesses which would be less risky for the girls and women flocking to these places to make money. This whole environment was a huge learning curve for me. It was the first time in my life I'd ever been exposed to anything like this, and it was eye opening. I remember one time sitting in one of these places with my colleague. She was conversing with a woman who was probably around 35 years old. This woman talked openly with us, told us she was HIV positive, and knew she would soon die. She admitted that she knew her work as a prostitute was extremely risky. Then she spoke, and I clearly recall her words. 'I can make more money having sex with truck drivers than I can by selling used clothes or selling cups of tea at a roadside stall. I'm saving the money I get and banking it so that my daughter doesn't have to do what I'm doing. I have had many of my friends die, and their daughters have been drawn into this business in order to survive. I don't want that to happen to my family.'

Life was tough for young girls and women in that environment. Family pressures brought them there to work in this life-threatening prostitution business and they had little choice other than to expose themselves to this risky way of making money. The male owners of the bars knew this; so, did many of the truck drivers, and they were quick to take advantage of it. It was a deeply troubling aspect of the work I was involved in. I have great admiration for my Tanzanian colleagues who continue, even today, to work in this extremely demanding field of health education.

Expelled from Tanzania

One day, Bruce came to me with devastating news. He'd had a phone call from the immigration department in Dar Es Salaam. He'd been told to inform me that my Tanzanian working visa had been cancelled. Consequently, I had to leave the country. This came as a huge shock to us both. I was devastated. Suddenly at risk in a foreign country, I packed a suitcase and was driven to the Kenyan border, and then on to Nairobi, a few hours' away, where a suitable hotel room was found for me. As I unpacked my few possessions, alone in my room, still in a state of shock, I began to wonder, what next? Bruce had assured me that he would get everything sorted; I had faith that he would. What had prompted them to revoke my visa? Thoughts raced through my mind. I suspected it was to do with my appointment to the position of HIV/AIDS Co-ordinator. As I understood it, some staff wanted this role to be given to a local person. Nothing was ever said officially, but the undercurrents were certainly there. So here I was in Kenya, an outcast from Tanzania, alone, wondering what I should do.

After a few days, I managed to shift from the hotel to a Christian guest house. This was certainly a much better environment for me. Many missionaries were passing through as they headed to different parts of Africa. A couple with whom I had been at Bible College turned up for a few days, and we had a great time together swapping stories. Every few days, I went to the World Vision office in Nairobi and helped where I could. However, the days ran into weeks and the uncertainty was weighing heavily on me. I didn't know what lay ahead; nor did I know how successful my study had been. It had been difficult enough undergoing the study for the exams; it had been even more demanding working on and submitting a thesis which I felt would probably be rejected because it wasn't written the right way.

Whenever a van arrived from Tanzania, it would bring my mail. As the time approached when I could expect to receive the results of my master's course in England, the arrival of the mail become even more important to me. Part of me was hanging out for the results; part of me feared what the outcome would be. It was an agonising wait.

The day a letter arrived

Finally, the day came when my results arrived. I sat with the letter from Brunel University in my hand. I hesitated, reluctant to open it. But I had to know, for better or for worse. I tore open the letter and stared at the contents in utter disbelief. I was stunned! Not only had I passed all my exams, but my dissertation had also passed with a B grade, a truly fantastic result! I couldn't believe it. Over the next few hours I kept reading the letter and re-reading it. Gradually, my success was sinking in; I was now Barbara Judith Walker, MSc in Medical Anthropology. My emotions were running riot: My friends had believed in me. My tutors had been so patient with me. My colleagues in Tanzania had supported me. And with God's help, and a large volume of blood, sweat and tears from me, I'd made it! I was desperate to tell my parents the good news. I waited until the time difference was right, and I rang them. On hearing my news, they were as amazed as I was, but also delighted, as they understood how difficult the study had been for me. The joy of my success lingered on. I was astonished, stunned, thrilled, amazed – there weren't enough words to describe how I was feeling. Incredibly I was now able to put MSc after my name; me, a person who had always struggled with reading and had done so poorly in School Certificate, only scraping through because of an amazing mark in History. I celebrated alone that night, sadly, as apart from me, the guesthouse was empty. A celebration party would have to come later. And sure enough, it did; a party and celebrations took place, some months later, when I returned to England for my graduation.

Somalia, here I come again

Meanwhile, I was still in Kenya, in exile. As far as my work was concerned, matters were now being taken in hand. While the Tanzanian visa issue was being sorted, World Vision needed a midwife to go to Somalia to run a course for Traditional Birth Attendants, and they planned to send me there to run it. I would be there for a couple of weeks and this course would take place in a new location for me – the town of Baidoa, in the southwest. Arrangements were made, and I flew off in a small plane from Nairobi. After a short flight, the plane landed at an airport in Southern Somalia, where, as I'd come to expect, there were no customs or immigration services.

Instead, a pickup truck loaded with men carrying AK-47 assault rifles drove right up to the plane to pick up passengers. There to meet me was a colleague with a local driver and four armed guards. I was shown into the back seat of the pickup truck and a couple of AK-47s were lifted from the seat and placed on the floor. I wasn't sure if they were loaded or not. I didn't really want to know. They took me to a house surrounded by a high, solid fence with barbed wire around the top, where I was shown to my room. Although basic, it had the necessities, so it was okay. Meanwhile the house girls were well under way with arrangements for lunch. Outside, on the corners of the fence were four towers occupied by armed guards, which, I was told, were on alert to spot any enemies.

As the days passed, I watched the guards taking turns at standing in the towers to make sure that no-one was coming to harm us. When they weren't on watch, they delighted in cleaning their guns, assembling them and then re-assembling them. They offered to teach me how to clean a gun, but I declined. I didn't think it would look so good on my CV in the future. I spent time with my colleague finding out what she wanted me to do, and we made plans for the course, which was to start in two days' time. The TBAs (Traditional Birth Attendants) from the surrounding area began to arrive and settle in until the day of the course arrived. After the welcomes and introductions, which took most of the morning, the teaching and sharing times began, assisted by a skilled interpreter. We were fortunate to have a model of the pelvis and a baby doll, so I was able to illustrate some basic anatomy to the TBAs. From the looks on their faces, this was something very new to them. Over the next few days, as stories were shared and teaching took place, there was much laughter and enjoyment. At the end of the course there was plenty of singing as each woman came forward to receive her certificate. Early next morning these women returned to their homes to continue their work as Traditional Birth Attendants, hopefully remembering something of what they had been taught.

The day I just wanted to die

After ten days in the excessively hot climate of Somalia, I woke up early one morning feeling extremely unwell. For the next few hours, I spent my time rushing to the toilet and vomiting my heart out. As dawn broke, the vomiting got so bad that I called out to my colleague who had been asleep in the next room. As she entered the room, she could clearly see I was in bad shape. She quickly called one of her co-workers who was a nurse. The nurse arrived and examined me. He said, 'Barbara, I think you need some intravenous fluids urgently.' He went back to his house and returned with the equipment needed. He then had several attempts to try and get a drip in, without success. He took my blood pressure, and by the look on his face I knew that things were not looking good. By then some of the Somali staff had arrived, and they were talking amongst themselves. I felt ghastly. I just wanted to see my Mum, and then die! A decision was made: One of the Somali staff would go to the local hospital and see if they could find a doctor and get him to come and see me. By now I was feeling so low that I didn't really care what happened. Continuing to vomit, I was in a such a weakened state that I couldn't even manage to walk to the toilet. Dignity was long gone by the time the Somali staff member returned. No doctors had been available, but he'd brought with him an anaesthetic technician skilled in putting in drips. After two attempts he got the drip in and the intravenous fluid began to flow. After a few hours, my colour improved, and my blood pressure rose. My colleagues contacted World Vision in Nairobi and it was agreed that they would get me on the flight out of Somalia later that day.

That same afternoon, with four litres of intravenous fluid inside me, I was placed on a skinny mattress in the pickup truck and driven to the airport and right up to the plane parked on the tarmac. Picking up the mattress, the Somali staff carried me into the plane, and placed the mattress on the floor between the two rows of seats. Six other passengers came on board and they had to climb over me to get to their seats.

The pilot informed me that there was a large green bucket by my feet, there, he said, should I need to use it. Everyone on board the plane could sympathise with me; all aid workers have had similar experiences. After the pilot gave the safety talk, we took off. It was a couple of hours to Nairobi and the pilot said he would try and avoid the bumps as I was the only passenger not wearing a seat belt. In the meantime, I was trying desperately to hang on, and not use the bucket. When we did go through a few bumps I bounced up and down a bit; no good for someone trying not to disgrace herself! When we landed in Nairobi, I was transferred to a medical clinic to get checked out. I assured them that I was now fine and just wanted to go to bed and sleep. World Vision had arranged for me to stay in a hotel, so I was taken there and assisted to sign in. As I was completing the form, I heard two familiar voices and turned around to see my two Swedish friends, Anders and Birgitta from the Mission Farm in Mpownge in Zambia, who were also signing in. What a wonderful surprise! It was hugging all round! I hadn't seen them since I had left Zambia; they had remained in Zambia and were now on their way home. We checked into our rooms and after we had all rested, I joined them for dinner (not that I could eat anything). While they ate, I drank lemonade, and thoroughly enjoyed catching up with old friends.

The next morning, I was feeling so much better. After breakfast my friends left to catch their flight home and I got a taxi to the World Vision office. On my arrival at the office, I was informed that my visa had been re-issued. I was free to return to Tanzania, which I did. Over the next few months there were significant changes. Bruce and his family left, and a new director was appointed. I was also considering my future, and spent much time thinking about possibilities, and praying to discern God's will for this next phase of my missionary service. Where would God take me next?

The closing of one door, the opening of another

Word came through that there was a potential position in Mozambique with World Vision, overseeing the health projects in the Tete Region of that country. I was invited to fly down and speak with the staff in the capital, Maputo, about this position. The interview was successful, and I was appointed to the position. I flew back to Tanzania to say goodbye to the staff there. It saddened me to have to say goodbye to some of the staff whom I had got to know so well over the last few years. I had learnt so much from them and they had been so patient with me and my lack of ability to learn Swahili. Yet, there was joy to come; I headed back to England for a few weeks of holiday. There I was able to attend my graduation ceremony.

Brunel University graduation day

My graduation day was truly amazing. Dressed in an academic gown, hood and mortarboard, and in the presence of my fellow students, staff and all their families and friends, I was overjoyed that I had made it. When my name was called out, I walked across that stage hardly daring to believe that it was true. It was for me a real miracle. So many people had believed in me, encouraging me to start the course when it had first been suggested to me. I was also immensely grateful to those who had supported me financially. Repeatedly, I gave thanks to God, who had journeyed with me through the whole course, and who continues to accompany me in what I do. I was delighted that some of my friends could be there to support me, though I regretted that none of my family could. It had all been such a huge challenge, both the academic work and the field work, including that day when I stood on the bridge on the Rwandan border, a gruelling day I will never forget.

My friends Sheila and Roger Derbridge originally from Liverpool, now living in Woking outside London, held a graduation party for me a few days later in their beautiful grounds. Speeches were made, food was eaten, and drinks flowed, and yes, a few tears were shed. Despite everything, including the struggle with dyslexia, the struggles I had, and still have, with reading, I was now Barbara, M.Sc. It was a miracle. It truly was.

My graduation euphoria was somewhat diminished by the next challenge I was facing. The position in Mozambique now required me go to Portugal, where I would be learning to speak Portuguese. With my persistent lack of success at learning languages, this was not a challenge I was looking forward to. I headed to Lisbon, wondering just how the next few weeks were going to unfold.

39. Three Weeks to Learn Portuguese: Yeah, Right!

With some trepidation, I flew to Portugal where I was to undertake a three-week course learning Portuguese. As you have gathered reading my story, I am certainly not a linguist, and I already considered this an impossible task. I arrived in Lisbon, found the accommodation that had been booked for me, and the next day I walked to the language school, which was close to the hotel. The language course was intensive, with classes running from Monday to Friday, and my progress was extremely slow. I happened to meet an Australian at the language school, who was heading to Angola, (also Portuguese speaking), with World Vision. It was good to have someone from 'Downunder' who could guide me around

Lisbon. He was nearing the end of his three-week course, and we were able to spend seven days together. Having another English-speaking person around was some comfort.

My teachers provided one-on-one teaching, showing incredible patience with my faltering attempts at using the language. They spent hours trying to encourage me as I wrestled with the unfamiliar sounds and words that made no sense to me. They encouraged me to explore the beautiful city of Lisbon in the evenings and weekends, and to use my Portuguese with the locals. One day in the early stages of the course my very patient language teacher said to me, 'Barbara, the staff have been discussing your language learning and we're wondering if you have ever been tested for dyslexia. After observing you over the last three weeks, we feel you may be struggling because of this condition.'

The aim of the course was for the students to have enough basic Portuguese language to build on once they got to the country to which they had been assigned. Each student had to prove this; on the last day at the language school, the students were expected to deliver a five-minute speech on what their plans were once they had left the course. For me, this was a huge mountain to climb. I certainly wasn't well equipped enough to complete this task. It was decided that an easier plan was needed for me, given my dyslexia. It would be acceptable for me to learn my small speech and recite it off by heart before the teachers. My speech would include a couple of sentences in which I would say my name, where I was from, and what I would be doing when I got to Mozambique.

The teachers worked hard with me, keen to see me succeed. Despite feeling immensely frustrated at my own shortcomings, and anxious about whether I would succeed, on the day of the graduation I did manage to say my short speech in Portuguese. Believe me, I pushed myself to the limit. My teachers were delighted. And I felt overwhelming relief. For my hard work I was given a small glass of port to celebrate this momentous event. I had a couple of ports that day! I felt so proud of what I'd been able to achieve.

Although I found the course in Lisbon very hard, I was pleased that someone had finally put their finger on what had been plaguing me all my life. It was a relief that the elephant in the room had been acknowledged even if it had taken over forty years to be named. Dyslexia wasn't something people talked about when I was a kid; I just knew I was very slow and struggled with reading. But it hadn't stopped me completing my nursing and midwifery training, Bible College training, or my master's degree in Medical Anthropology. After years of wondering why I found reading so hard and why I was so useless at trying to understand and learn foreign languages (highlighted by all those language tests I had failed in New Zealand years earlier), my suspicions were finally confirmed in Lisbon all those years later, at the age of 45.

I felt a relief at this, and that the course was over, but was fully aware that my next assignment to manage a health project in Mozambique wasn't going to be easy. However, I was ready for the challenge, knowing that I would give this new role my best, as I always did. Little did I know what was going to unfold that Saturday morning, while I drank a cup of coffee, and suddenly heard a knock on my door.

40. Coming Home

I am safe

It was 1996, and I had just been through the most trying period of my life. My time in Mozambique had ended; I was able to leave the country safely, though not untouched, as I was still quite affected by what had happened. As the plane circled Auckland and came into land, I looked out of the window and saw the grass, the simple houses and the welcoming airport. My eyes filled with tears. I was safe. I was home. Quietly, I sat in my seat and silently prayed, and thanked God that I was back in my country and very soon would be hugging family and friends. I was exhausted in every way. I had no idea what the next few weeks, months or years would hold, but I knew that God knew; I trusted Him, that when the time was right, things would fall into place.

Returning to New Zealand in 1996 was hard. No one spoke about conditions such as Post-Traumatic Stress Syndrome. Kiwis were expected to just get on with their lives, regardless of any trauma, and let others get on with theirs. So, I was extremely fortunate to have some special friends who understood and were there for me, listening to me and supporting me as best they could. A number of these friends had either worked overseas in similar situations, or they had been out to visit me in the field, so they had some idea of what it was like. I am eternally grateful to them, and to God for providing them. Despite this support, I can remember many times when I would go for a walk with friends, and if I heard any noise, I would start, and quickly turn around to make sure no one was following me. Clearly, it wasn't going to be quick or easy to leave Mozambique behind, despite the kilometres between us.

A time of reflection

When I first went overseas to a crisis in 1979, Stanley Mooneyham, the International Director of World Vision at the time, spoke one Sunday morning at Valley Road Baptist church in Auckland, where I attended. He shared this message with us that day:

> 'There are many stories in the Bible where Jesus ministered to one person at a time. I am sure while he was ministering to that one person in the crowd, others would be struggling with their lives and some probably even died. That needs to be your model, hard though it may be.'

It was indeed a hard lesson, and a difficult model to follow. Many times, while I was overseas, there were just so many people who needed immediate attention, but, like Jesus, I could only seek to help one person at a time. Yes, I know others died when they didn't get the help they needed. That's the tragedy. But gut-wrenching as it may be, we had to come to terms with the fact that we couldn't help everyone. Safely back in New Zealand, I was spending a lot of time reflecting on the various situations, places, and people I had met while away from this place. In all the places I'd worked, I had certainly sought to do my best, and I believe that I did. Looking back, perhaps there were some situations I could have handled better, but hindsight is a fine thing. My re-entry to New Zealand was a time of serious introspection, of searching inside myself. It was also a time to begin looking forward, wondering what the future would bring.

Reacquaintances

Although my family and friends gave me a warm welcome, there were people in my family who were no longer around, as both of my grandmothers had died while I was overseas. Friends had also died, and I appreciated when others took me to their graves so that I could pay my respects. My parents and my siblings were especially relieved that I was back home in one piece, but my nieces and nephews didn't really know who I was. They had heard of this person called Aunty Barbara, who appeared in the newspapers, and in radio and TV interviews. She would visit occasionally, never forgetting to bring them gifts, and then she would disappear again to reappear later, even years later. Even though I was so distant from them for many years, I am extremely proud of all my nieces and nephews, and the ever-increasing number of great-nieces and great-nephews. My return to New Zealand gave me time to get to know them all better through more regular contact. It was a special thrill when my brother Philip and his wife Christine asked me to be Godmother to their son, Jack Walker. I have taken great delight in following Jack's journey through life, watching him grow into a very special young man.

Re-entry

I also went through a kind of reverse culture shock during my first-year home. I wasn't expecting this, and it took me somewhat by surprise. I thought I would just return to New Zealand and slot back in, but New Zealand had changed, and so had I. When people talked about the Springbok Rugby tour riots of 1981 or Rogernomics, I hadn't a clue what they were talking about. In fact, so much had changed since I had left New Zealand in 1975, I felt like a foreigner. I was floundering and it was hard.

At times I felt quite ignorant! Things like going to the bank were a challenge. I was frequently told by the bank staff to use the 'hole in the wall.' 'The what?' I would ask... I remember visiting the 'Red Shed,' one of the very popular Warehouse stores that had sprung up all over New Zealand; it sold everything! I just walked up and down the aisles, looking in astonishment at all the goods one could buy.

Reflections

Having been overseas working as a nurse midwife in such demanding and challenging situations for nearly twenty years, and working far beyond my New Zealand Nursing Council and New Zealand Midwifery Council scope of practice, I wondered where I could possibly fit in if I continued to work as a nurse and midwife here. If I carried out some of the procedures, I had undertaken in the countries I'd worked in, I would be struck off the registers and probably fined heavily as well. I'd developed a range of skills that were not only unique to me, they were part of me, and I knew that I wouldn't be able to use them here in New Zealand. I had worked not only as a midwife and nurse; I had worked more often as a medical, surgical or obstetric registrar, a dentist, an anaesthetist or an eye surgeon, diagnosing, prescribing, even operating. I had also done the job of X-ray technician at times in Zambia, and I had developed skills in car mechanics, plumbing and carpentry. (I had also gained driving skills which a rally driver would be proud of!)

I had dealt with the international press, film crews, and celebrities. I had been on assignments that saw me working with challenging government officials, alongside United Nations personnel, in different non-government organisations, with people of so many different cultures and beliefs. Who would want to employ such a uniquely skilled person? Where could I possibly fit?

Knowing I had to find work, I spent some time in the World Vision New Zealand office and was offered a position in Rwanda. After much thought and even more prayer, I declined it. I didn't think it was a good idea to go from the traumatic events of Mozambique into another stressful situation in Rwanda. For me, that was a watershed moment. The fact that I would never go back overseas as a nurse-midwife aid worker was my new reality.

About 18 months after I came home, I was offered counselling. I went to see a counsellor who I had known prior to going overseas. When we finally got together, she asked me, 'Barbara, what have you been up to since we met back in the 1970s when you were nursing in Auckland?'

'How long have you got?' I asked.

'About an hour this session,' She replied. So, I gave her a brief outline of the last 20 years; her only comment was: 'Wow.' She was surprised I hadn't been to see her sooner. I eventually had a few sessions with her, which were helpful for me.

I had thought long and hard about what to do workwise when I came home. I wanted to find somewhere in New Zealand where I could learn from a community and be of some assistance to them through sharing what I'd learnt through years spent in disaster and development work, and from my studies in Medical Anthropology. Set on working back in New Zealand, I considered several possible roles and applied for positions in Ruatoria, East Cape Region and at Rawene Hospital in the Hokianga in Northland. I was interviewed for the position with Hauora Hokianga.

The Hauora Hokianga Model had a practical grass roots approach which was to empower local communities to address their community's health needs. Over the years, many nurses, doctors and other health professionals have been attracted to work in the community in Northland. When I heard about what they were doing up there I thought that maybe this is where God wanted me next. I applied, and in 1997 I was appointed the First Community Health Manager for Hauora Hokianga

It was an interesting time for me in Northland, and I learnt a lot. I am particularly grateful to my colleagues and the community who made me feel welcome in this special, although at times challenging, environment. I was grateful to my sister Jillian and her partner Brian Potiki (who had lived in the area at one time and were Te Reo Maori speakers), who, along with their young daughter Hira, introduced me to the to the local community at a very moving Pōwhiri (a traditional Maori welcome). This experience brought back so many memories of being welcomed into different communities around the world. This time, I was back in my own country, but I was now living in a very different culture; as a white person of European background, I was suddenly in the minority in my own country. Having struggled to learn other languages all around the world, I tried desperately to learn Te Reo, which was widely spoken in that area. Predictably, it was too hard for me, and I regret to this day my inability to master it. My role within the Health Trust was to oversee the community health work, including community mental health, community nurses, dental workers and the home helpers who assisted people in their homes.

I enjoyed working with the staff and learnt a lot from them. It was certainly a divine appointment for me, as a lot of the work I had been involved in overseas was working at the grass roots level, listening and empowering local people. Issues of water, housing and communicable diseases were often talked about and solutions discussed, which was like my work in many of the places that I had worked in overseas. There were a lot of challenges working in the Hokianga; the isolation, the poverty, growing unemployment, cannabis, but there was also a wonderful community spirit and many committed people who wanted to make a difference. During my time there, parts of the Hokianga experienced a devastating flood, with a huge loss of roads, houses, and basic infrastructure. It was a privilege to work alongside the people as they rallied around and supported each other. Help came in from around the country, but it was the local leaders supported by their people who worked tirelessly to rebuild their communities.

The staff who worked for Hokianga Health provided a wonderful community-based health program, and for me being part of that brought back many memories of my work with communities in Africa. Another similarity is the way that the community nurses work hard to ensure that where possible, terminally ill patients who wanted to spend their final days in their homes could do so, surrounded by the family, with daily visits from the nurses. The hospital in Rawene, where I was based, had its own marae and many meetings, both formal and informal took place there. I also had the opportunity to attend several Treaty of Waitangi workshops, which was something new for me, and they certainly helped me to understand something of the history of my own country. It was often a steep learning curve, but one which I was very grateful to be involved in.

It was also good to be home, as my parents' health was changing as they became older. My mum was not experiencing good health. Being in New Zealand, I was able to support both her and Dad and to give back to them something of what they had given to me all their lives. My mum had had some major surgical events while I was overseas, and I am forever grateful that I was able to fly home at those times from some of the farthest places in the world to be with her and Dad. This time I wouldn't be flying away again. It was timely.

In 1998, my Dad came up to spend a few days with me while I was living in the Hokianga, while my Aunt Philippa Swanson went and stayed with Mum in Whakatane, as she wasn't well enough to make the journey north. Word came through late one afternoon that Mum had suffered a massive heart attack and was in a critical condition in Whakatane Hospital. Distraught, we managed to get word to two of my siblings, Philip, and Jenny Tapsell, who were thankfully able to get to see her before she died. Dad and I left the Hokianga straight away. I drove all though the night to get to Whakatane, conscious of Dad's grief at not being there with Mum when she died, and my own grief at this loss of a much-loved parent. Choking back my tears, I managed to get us there safely, with other family members arriving the following day.

Together we planned the funeral, which Dad had asked me to take. Although I had led and taken part in funerals for colleagues overseas, conducting my Mum's funeral service was completely different. It was an honour, but it was also heart-rending. With God's gracious help and the loving support of my family and friends from which I drew strength, we were able to give Mum a special service. Mum was so proud of all her children. We would miss her so much. I was so pleased that I could be there with my family at this sad time, and that we could be there for each other.

In 2010 I was with my sister Sue when dad passed away at Whakatane Hospital, other siblings arrived at the hospital a short time later. Working together we organised his funeral which I had the privilege to lead. Having mourned two of my grandmothers while I was working overseas, I was so pleased that I was back in New Zealand when both my parents died. At such sad times it was comforting for all of us siblings to be together and support each other along with other family members and friends.

41. A Time for Recognition

Fellow of the College of Nurses of Aotearoa New Zealand

I was thrilled when, in 1999, the College of Nurses of Aotearoa honoured me by making me a Fellow of the College of Nurses of Aotearoa New Zealand for 'having demonstrated professional excellence and leadership in nursing.'

The fellowship category of membership is available to nurses who have earned recognition for their outstanding contribution to nursing in a field. To this day, I don't know who nominated me for this award as I received a letter from the College out of the blue, asking me if I would accept. Once again, I was mindful of the support I'd received that made my achievements possible. I felt the award honoured those others in my life too, especially the nurses I worked alongside in so many countries; in New Zealand and around the world. My first ward sister at Greenlane Hospital who gave me that first nursing report would have smiled if she knew that I had been given this award.

And yet another award soon came my way. After my own presentation to a regional Rotary Conference in 1997, I was honoured with the Jean Harris International Award, 'in recognition of outstanding service to the development and progress of women in society.' What an honour! As I received this prestigious award, I wanted to acknowledge the local staff in the countries where I had worked. Without their support, patience and willingness to act as my interpreters, I would not have been able to carry out my role.

New Zealand Queen's Birthday Honours, 2000

One day in early 2000, I received an official letter from Government House informing me that Her Majesty the Queen had awarded me a QSO (Queen's Service Order) for my work overseas and in the Hokianga. I was absolutely blown away and couldn't believe what I was reading. Tears spilled down my cheeks as I read and reread the letter. I was asked to tell no one, and to expect contact from the media just prior to the Queen's Birthday weekend, when the names on the honours list would be released.

I wrote back saying I would be honoured to accept the award. At my family-only event in Auckland a couple of days before the media announcement, I shared my news with the family. There were tears and delight, but I was sad that my Mum didn't get to hear the news. Mum and Dad were both extremely supportive of me, and Mum had been an active participant for many years in the annual World Vision 40 Hour Famine fund-raiser, supporting World Vision in her own way. Despite their initial hesitation when I first went overseas, they were very proud of their second daughter, and indeed of all their children.

Official letters came, informing me of the arrangements for the presentation of my QSO, and dates on which ceremonies would be held. I chose my birthday, the 9th of August 2000, and duly arrived at Government House along with my Dad, two siblings, and a good nursing friend. We all got dressed up, and I had bought a very expensive outfit for this once-in-a-lifetime experience, but without the long gloves or the hat that were once worn on such formal occasions! It was a memorable day, mixing with other Kiwis and their families who were being recognised for the work they had done, in New Zealand and around the world.

My turn came. I walked forward to receive my award. The Governor General, the Rt Hon Sir Michael Hardie Boyes, shared a few words with me and I with him, then I returned to my seat. As we all stood for the singing of the National Anthem, I for one had tears in my eyes.

As I stood there, I thought of all the national staff members in the many countries where I had worked, who had been so patient as I struggled with their language, but working in partnership, we sought to make a difference, and in some places, we did. I thought of the traditional birth attendants, from whom I had learnt so much, and who gave me the title of this book, *Purple Hands*; they who are still out there in very primitive conditions, possibly with no water, but perhaps delivering babies using their very skilled, possibly purple hands. I thought of those who had lost their lives in the camps, and those who had made it to safety. I thought of those New Zealanders who had given financial support to the various agencies which were seeking to make a difference. I thought of my family and friends who had stood by me and supported me with their love and prayers over the years I was away. But most of all I was grateful to God, who'd called me by name all those years ago, who had been there with me every day, through the good times as well as the tough times, the times when I was so scared, or so sick, and yes, the lonely times. It was a momentous day, a day in which I was so proud to be a New Zealander and a citizen of God's world.

I was delighted on the 30th of December 2017 when my sister Jill was awarded a Queen Service Medal (QSM) for services to art and children. A special time of celebration for our family. My parents would have been so thrilled.

The Margarette Golding Award

In 2012, I was also honoured to be the recipient of the International Inner Wheel Margarette Golding Award for highly commendable personal service, in recognition of my 'outstanding medical and missionary care of people, both in the difficult conditions of war ravaged countries in Africa and subsequently in New Zealand,' generously granted to me by the Inner Wheel Club of Ahuriri Napier. These wonderful honours always made me feel humble and proud, but I still felt like just a small-town Kiwi girl, who just happened to be called to do God's work.

Back to my roots

After three years, I left the Hokianga. I had given my best to this special community and, when a position came up to manage a Health Trust in Milton Otago, I felt it was time to return to my roots in the South Island. While living in Milton, I discovered that my great-grandmother had been born there; it was special to be back where some of my ancestors came from. I managed the trust for three years and, although I enjoyed the management side, I struggled with the nursing side. It was hard adapting to a health system that was so very different from what I'd been used to for so long overseas.

Although I had done a 'return to nursing' course at the local polytech, I felt restricted in what I could and could not do. There were so many new things to learn: new medications, a huge variety of dressings for different types of wounds and ulcers, new drugs, and so many rules, procedures and restrictions. Over the last twenty years, this practical Kiwi nurse midwife had used what she had; torn up sheets for bandages, papaya to assist in cleaning wounds, gentian violet and hydrogen peroxide as antiseptics, and recycled gloves, when we were lucky enough to have them. I was used to the most limited medications and even more limited choice of dressings. Now I was back in a First World country with so many choices of medications and dressings and everything else that I found it all very overwhelming.

Rebirth of the call to ordination

I began to wonder what God's plans were for me. I had been a nurse and midwife for many years, and I had loved it, especially my years working overseas. I wanted to stay in the medical arena, but I didn't want to nurse for the rest of my working life. As I prayed and thought long and hard, a small spark which was buried deep inside my heart began to glow.

Over several years, I had talked with clergy friends about the possibility of ordination. One of these was Lord Coggan, a former Archbishop of Canterbury, whom I had got to know while on leave in the United Kingdom, and during his and his wife's visits to Bannu. However, I had shelved the idea of ordination, feeling the time was not right.

During my time in Milton, I often thought about ordination and talked to friends who had gone into ordained ministry. The hospital chaplaincy attracted me, and I began to consider heading in that direction. I felt that so much of my background would lend itself to this calling: my nursing and medical background, my years of cross cultural experiences, working alongside people of different faith groups, my interest in people (especially those facing tough, life-challenging experiences), and the ability to work under huge pressure, often with limited staff and resources in short supply. This realisation was to lead me into the next stage in my Christian journey.

The urge was getting stronger and I felt it was something God was calling me to. During a trip to Te Anau with Penny Jamieson, then Bishop of Dunedin, she asked me, 'Barbara, what are you going to do when you finish nursing?' I told her that I felt God was leading me into hospital chaplaincy. She said, 'You need to get ordained.'

After more prayer and conversations with trusted friends, I was convinced by a deep inner feeling that ordination, followed by hospital chaplaincy, was the path I was being led down. I was excited, but also apprehensive as I started on this new journey. At the time, I was in Milton managing the health trust, but soon after, moved into Dunedin to manage a retirement home for the Salvation Army. There, I regularly attended St Matthew's Anglican church.

Over several years while living in the Diocese of Dunedin, I was guided through the path towards ordination. This involved training in a variety of aspects of becoming an Anglican priest. At times I found the extra study, watching and working alongside clergy, plus interviews and more interviews and regular supervision, quite overwhelming. But God's call on my life to take this path was very strong, and with His empowerment, and support from friends and local clergy, I continued. The words I chose as mine so long ago, 'The one who calls you is faithful, and He will do it'(1 Thessalonians 5:24), continually rang in my ears and strengthened my faith in God and in this decision.

Eventually, the time came for me to be ordained as a deacon in the Anglican Church. In June 2003, family members from all over New Zealand, parishioners from my home church St Matthew's, work colleagues and rest home residents I was managing all came together for this momentous event in St Paul's Cathedral in Dunedin. I felt truly blessed to have such wonderful support.

Ann Pollington, a friend from one of my link parishes in the United Kingdom, who supported me during my time in Pakistan all those years ago, flew to Dunedin and sang during the service; this was her gift to me. Nine months later, in 2004, I was ordained as a priest. I was now the Reverend Barbara Walker. This was also a very moving service, with the added highlight of being able to serve Holy Communion to family members, including my Dad.

It was such a joy when I was also able to attend my youngest sister Jenny Tapsell's ordination in St Paul's Cathedral in Dunedin in 2015. To have two children who are Anglican priests in the one family would have made my parents so proud.

42. 'Sister Barbara, You Still Haven't Learnt Urdu!'

Not long after I became ordained, I was able to contribute to the missions again when I moved to Auckland and worked for the New Zealand Church Missionary Society (NZCMS), recruiting and supporting the next generation who would go and work in many of the countries I had worked in previously. During this time, I had the privilege of revisiting the Pennell Memorial Hospital in Bannu. The headmaster of the Pennell High School drove to Islamabad to collect Mary, a kiwi teacher who was working into another area of Pakistan. Wearing traditional Pakistani dress, Mary and I arrived at the headmaster's home at the Pennell High School which shared a compound with the hospital.

As I got out of the vehicle, the first person I saw was a tall, handsome young man whom I had delivered many years earlier; he and his parents had come to greet me. After our initial greetings, they exclaimed, 'Sister Barbara, you still haven't learnt Urdu!' and we were taken on a tour of the beautiful new hospital and shown into a large room where staff had gathered. Garlands were placed around our necks and spontaneous singing began. My fluent Urdu-speaking friend Mary translated the speeches for me. Then it was my turn to greet those gathered and I expressed my delight at being back 'home' in Bannu. The hospital superintendent acknowledged the work I'd done, and then offered me a midwifery position which I gracefully declined. Then he asked, 'Sister Barbara, what can we do for you? You have done so much for us!' I thought for a minute and said, 'I would like to deliver a baby.' Everyone laughed. They recalled how Sister Barbara was always delivering babies, hundreds of babies. 'I'll see what we can do,' the superintendent said.

At 3.00 am the next morning we were woken by a knock on the door. Sleepily, I opened the door and an armed guard said there was a delivery case. Would I come? Dressing hurriedly, Mary and I were escorted across the road to the hospital delivery suite by the guards. Mary, a teacher, was excited, as she had never seen a baby being born.

The Pakistani midwife said the patient was in strong labour and having her first baby. Examining the woman, I noted the strength of her contractions and realised she should deliver within an hour or so. Memories of the hundreds of babies I'd delivered in this hospital came flooding back. The patient's contractions were getting stronger and soon she was ready to push. A few minutes later I had the joy of delivering a beautiful, healthy Afghan baby. I wrapped the newborn in a small blanket and handed her to the mother. But she turned her head away and refused to take the baby. What sadness!

The baby was a girl, and in Afghan society, boy babies are much preferred. Mary was delighted to hold the baby girl while I delivered the placenta. I handed the patient back and thanked the midwife and the patient for allowing me to deliver her baby. When we returned to our sleeping quarters, Mary and I prayed that this wee girl would be loved and cared for by her family. The next day we headed back to Islamabad. From there I flew back to New Zealand, leaving my colleague to continue her ministry in Pakistan. During my time with NZCMS, I visited New Zealand workers in Tanzania, Rwanda, Cambodia, Egypt (and other places I am not able to mention for security reasons). Life continued to unfold.

43. A New Direction

While working for NZCMS, I also travelled to Hastings, in Hawke's Bay, to speak to church groups about overseas missions. There, I met Drs Alison and John Kerr who hosted a colleague and me during our stay. They were wonderful hosts and we had many interesting conversations about missions. I spoke with Alison and John about my desire to become a hospital chaplain. Sometime later when I was visiting another part of New Zealand, John rang to tell me of the resignation of the coordinating hospital chaplain at the Hawke's Bay Fallen Soldiers' Memorial Hospital in Hastings and encouraged me to apply for the position. I applied, and the rest, as they say, is history. I commenced my new ministry on 9 February 2009. With my nursing and midwifery background and experience in working alongside people of many different cultures and religions, I know this is where God wants me to be. When I retire my hospital chaplaincy journey will be the topic for my second book, which I hope you will all be reading soon.

> 'What counts is not the mere fact that we have lived. It is what difference we have made to the lives of others that will determine the significance of the life we lead.'
>
> *Nelson Mandela*

Index

B
Bailey, Judy 180
Barratt-Boyes, Brian 26
Best-Walker, Christine 180
Bono 124
Briant, Dr Robin 44, 60

C
Coggan, Dr Ruth 92, 93, 96, 98, 100, 114, 125, 132
Coggan, Lady Jean 93
Coggan, Lord Donald 93, 198
Crombie, Kathy 83
cultural issues 48, 59, 114, 151
  female circumcision 62

D
de la Perrelle, Frank 18
de la Perrelle, Mabel 18, 22, 136
Derbridge, Roger 85, 88, 187
Derbridge, Sheila 85, 88, 187

G
Geldof, Bob 124

H
Hamlin, Dr Catherine 125
Hamlin, Dr Reginald 125
Hardie Boyes, Rt Hon Sir Michael 196
Holt, Rosemary 113

I
Inder, June 47
Inder, Peter 47, 48

J
Jamieson, Bishop Penny 199

K
Kerr, Dr Alison 202
Kerr, Dr John 202
Kippenberger, Carolyn (Kipp) 118, 124, 126, 127, 128, 129, 131, 136

M
Machel, Samora 9
Mandela, Nelson 202
McConchie, Bruce 15, 16, 165, 169
McConchie, Margaret 169
Moi, Daniel arap 56
Mondlane, Eduardo 9
Mooneyham, Stanley 50, 190
Mother Teresa 80
Myles, Maggie 100

N
New Zealand Church Missionary Society 95

P
Parker, Warren 89
Pennell, Dr Theodore 92
Pollington, Ann 199
Potiki, Brian 193
Potiki, Hira 193
Pot, Pol 39
Prentice, Colin 15
purple hands, reason for book title 64

S
Seasweep, international rescue ship 50, 52
Sims, Heather 31, 100
Swanson, Philippa 163, 194

T
Tapsell (nee Walker), Jennifer 20, 194, 200
Taylor, Richard 48
Thayer, Sheryl 17
trachoma, eye disease 67
traditional birth attendants, Somalia 62

W
Walker, Barbara
  aid agencies worked for
    Church Missionary Society United Kingdom 88
    Finnish mission, Kenya 137
    New Zealand Church Missionary Society 200
    Swedish Free Baptist Mission Board, Zambia 152
    World Vision 9, 10, 38, 40, 43, 85, 116, 165, 180, 183
  awards and recognition
    Fellow of the College of Nurses of Aotearoa New Zealand 195
    International Inner Wheel Margarette Golding Award 197
    Jean Harris International Award, Rotary 195
    Queen's Service Order (QSO) 196
  Christian faith 18
    1 Thessalonians 5:24 33, 199
    God's call 22, 24, 33, 36, 198
    Valley Road Baptist Church 31, 37
  early years
    Melville High School 23
    Millerton 19
    Mokoia 20
    Ohaupo 23
    Portland 21
    Riverton 18
  personal illnesses, conditions and treatment
    dehydration
      Kenya 56
      Somalia 185
    dengue fever, Thailand 46
    endometriosis, Pakistan 134
    hysterectomy 152
    typhoid, Pakistan 128
  places visited
    Ampipal, Nepal 83
    Chad border with Sudan 78
    El Genenia, Sudan 77
    Islamabad, Pakistan 90
    Nairobi, Kenya
      Norfolk Hotel bomb 72
    New Hebrides (Vanuatu) 28
    the Seychelles 74
  places worked in New Zealand
    Greenlane Hospital 23, 24, 53
    Hawke's Bay Fallen Soldiers' Memorial Hospital, Hastings 202
    Rawene Hospital, Hokianga 192
    St Helen's Hospital 30
    Wairoa Hospital 31
  places worked in other countries
    Baidoa, Somalia 183
    Bannu, Pakistan 87, 92, 127
      Pennell Memorial Hospital 90, 200
    Calcutta 80
    Ibnat, Ethiopia 116
    Kapedo Mission Hospital, Kenya 140
    Khao I Dang, Thailand 42, 48

Las Dhure, Somalia 55, 57
Mozambique 10
Mpongwe Mission Hospital, Zambia 154
Sakeo One Refugee Camp, Thailand 39
serious incidents
  car accident, Kenya 138
  death threat, Mozambique 11
  room burgled, Tanzania 169
Singapore 51
roles undertaken
  anaesthetist, Zambia 160
  carpentry 43
  Community Health Manager, Hauora, Hokianga 193
  dentist, Zambia 159
  district nurse, Tasmainia 36
  eye surgery
    Ethiopia 121
    Kenya 149
    Somalia 68
  HIV Aids Consultant, Tanzania 180
  HIV/AIDS trainer, Tanzania 165
  hospital chaplain, Hastings 202
  manager, health trust, Milton, Otago 197
  manager, Salvation Army retirement home, Dunedin 199
  matron, Kapedo mission hospital, Kenya 139
  midwife 62
  missionary nurse 29
  ordained deacon, Anglican Church 199
  ordained priest, Anglican Church 199
  parish sister for the Tasmanian Anglican Church 36
  plumber 66
  staff nurse 53
  technical manager, Ibnat, Ethiopia 121
training and study undertaken
  Bible college, Tasmania 32
  disaster management 85
  graduation as New Zealand Registered Midwife 31
  graduation as New Zealand Registered Nurse 27
  Liverpool School of Tropical Medicine 85
  Masters degree, Medical Anthropology, Brunel University, London 164, 171, 183
  Murree language school, Pakistan 94
  nursing training 24
  Tasmania 32
Walker, Frank 18, 21, 47, 194
Walker, Jack 191
Walker, Jillian 20, 193, 197
Walker, Marie 18, 21, 47, 194
Walker, Philip 21, 47, 180, 194
Walker, Ruby 50
Walker, Susan 22, 195
Walker, Vaughan 18
Werner, David 60
Wood (nee Walker), Wendy 19, 127

www.ingramcontent.com/pod-product-compliance
Lightning Source LLC
Chambersburg PA
CBHW072006070526
44583CB00015B/1360